A Pocket Guide to Clinical Decision-making in Wound Management

Other titles available from Wounds UK include:

Honey: A modern wound management product edited by Richard White, Rose Cooper and Peter Molan

Essential Wound Management: An introduction for undergraduates edited by David Gray, Pam Cooper and John Timmons

Wound Healing: A systematic approach to advanced wound healing and management edited by David Gray and Pam Cooper

Wounds UK — The Directory, 2007 edited by Richard White and Clare Morris

Trauma and Pain in Wound Care edited by Richard White and Keith Harding

Paediatric Skin and Wound Care edited by Richard White and Jacqueline Denyer

This book is supported by an unrestricted educational grant from ConvaTec Limited. ConvaTec had no editorial control over the content of this text. The comments and views expressed are those of the authors only and do not necessarily reflect those of ConvaTec.

®Hydrofiber is a registered trade mark of E.R. Squibb & Sons, L.L.C., ConvaTec is an authorised user.

A Pocket Guide to Clinical Decision-making in Wound Management

edited by

Sue Bale and David Gray

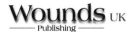

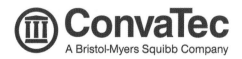

Wounds UK Publishing, Wounds UK Limited, Suite 3.1, 36 Upperkirkgate, Aberdeen AB10 1BA

British Library Cataloguing-in-Publication Data
A catalogue record is available for this book

© Wounds UK Limited 2006
ISBN 0-9549193-4-3

Printed in the UK by Cromwell Press, Trowbridge, Wiltshire

CONTENTS

LIST OF CONTRIBUTORS

Sue Bale is Associate Director of Nursing, Gwent Healthcare NHS Trust, South Wales.

Martyn Butcher is Clinical Nurse Specialist, Tissue Viability, Derriford Hospital, Plymouth.

Madeleine Flanagan is Principal Lecturer, School of Continuing Professional Development, University of Hertfordshire.

Jacqui Fletcher is Principal Lecturer, School of Nursing and Midwifery, University of Hertfordshire.

INTRODUCTION

There are many choices available for accessing information on how best to care for patients with wounds. Much has been written about wound healing and wound care in books and journals, associations have been formed, clinical nurse specialist practice has been developed, websites have been set up, and a broad range of educational courses are available, from MSc programmes through to day courses. Many of these are targeted at specialists that need advanced, detailed, and in depth information to meet their requirements.

This pocket guide provides nurses working at the bedside with a framework for making clinical decisions and taking a structured approach to wound care. It uses the Wound Progression Model as the framework, where wound care is mapped from the underlying causes, to wound bed condition, treatment aims and treatment options. The text provides practical advice to guide clinical decision-making, based on research findings and clinical guidelines.

The reader will find that the first chapter comprehensively, but succinctly, covers the causes of acute and chronic wounds, presenting the pathologies related to common wound types. *Chapter 2* provides a guide to progressing the wound through the healing process, using the Wound Progression Model and the Wound Healing Continuum. Wound symptoms are a frequent clinical challenge and *Chapter 3* explores the management of odour, exudate, pain and bleeding. The final chapter draws the earlier ones together, presenting flow diagrams to guide clinical decision-making. Each flow diagram is accompanied by a patient case scenario to illustrate how they work in practice.

Sue Bale FRCN, PhD, BA, RGN, NDN, RHV, PG Dip, Dip N
Associate Director of Nursing (R&D)
Gwent Healthcare NHS Trust
South Wales
March, 2006

WOUND PROGRESSION MODEL

CAUSE	PROGRESSION TO HEALING	SYMPTOM MANAGEMENT
BEFORE DECIDING ON ANY TREATMENT PLAN, AN UNDERSTANDING OF THE WOUND'S CAUSE IS REQUIRED	THE PRESENCE OF NECROTIC, SLOUGHY TISSUE, OR INFECTION, CAN DELAY THE PROGRESSION TO HEALING	THE MANAGEMENT OF SYMPTOMS ASSOCIATED WITH WOUNDS SUCH AS THOSE LISTED BELOW CAN BE FACILITATED BY THE CORRECT SELECTION OF PRODUCTS

CAUSE

- LEG ULCER
- DIABETIC FOOT ULCER
- PRESSURE ULCER
- BURN
- SURGICAL WOUND
- TRAUMATIC WOUND

PROGRESSION TO HEALING

REMOVE NECROSIS	REMOVE SLOUGH	MANAGE INFECTION

PROMOTE GRANULATION

DELAYED HEALING, KICK-START HEALING

PROMOTE EPITHELIALISATION

SYMPTOM MANAGEMENT

- ODOUR
- PAIN
- BLEEDING
- EXUDATE
  >HIGH   >MEDIUM   >LOW

CHAPTER 1

WOUND PATHOLOGIES: CAUSES OF ACUTE AND CHRONIC WOUNDS

Madeleine Flanagan and Jacqui Fletcher

Wound assessment is a complex process that helps to determine wound aetiology and the progress of healing over time. The holistic management of any patient and their wounds depends on a logical and structured approach to care. The Wound Progression Model suggests three main themes:

- identify the cause
- progress the wound to healing
- look after the patient.

In identifying the cause of the wound, the underlying aetiology must be diagnosed. This is considered, together with any intrinsic or extrinsic factors that have been identified, as part of the holistic assessment which may perpetuate or prolong the healing. Progressing the wound to healing involves appropriate management of the wound, the patient and the care environment, alongside a good working relationship with the patient, family or carers. Looking after the patient should flow throughout the care delivery, and includes addressing issues identified by the patient, who may have different priorities to the care giver. Good education is also essential for the patient to make well-informed decisions.

During normal acute wound healing, a series of regulated molecular events prepares the wound for repair and wound closure. However, this process of molecular and cellular control is impaired in chronic wounds, resulting in a delay in, or failure to achieve, complete healing (Schultz *et al*, 2003). Chronic wounds are characterised by a fixed, persistent inflammatory state, abnormal deposition of the extracellular matrix (ECM), and failure to epithelialise. The prolonged inflammatory response is caused by elevated levels of pro-inflammatory cytokines and decreased growth factor activity. Healing of chronic wounds is further complicated by local and systemic factors, such as infection, ischaemia, concomitant diseases, eg. diabetes, and drug therapies, such as glucocorticoids.

Acute wounds can be defined as following the normal healing process in a defined time-frame without complications, and are classified according to type of injury, eg. surgical, traumatic (Bates-Jensen and Wethe, 1998). In contrast, the normal process of healing is disrupted in chronic wounds at one or more points in the phases of haemostasis, inflammation, proliferation, and remodelling, resulting in delayed healing or a failure to heal (Price and Enoch, 2004). Chronic wounds are classified according to their underlying pathology, eg. pressure ulcers, venous leg ulcers.

Chronic wound fluid has been shown to delay proliferation of endothelial cells, fibroblasts and keratinocytes. Increased proteases break down angiogenic factors so that development of healthy granulation tissue is disrupted (Chen and Abatangelo, 1999). Chronic wound fluid contains high levels of pro-inflammatory cytokines that inhibit growth of skin fibroblasts, which have a central role in healing as they stimulate angiogenesis and epithelialisation, and produce extracellular proteins (Agren *et al*, 1999).

The production and activity of matrix metalloproteinases (MMPs) is tightly controlled in acute wounds. Matrix metalloproteinases play an important role in intracellular signalling by stabilising growth factors and regulating the structure of the ECM. Levels of MMPs are greatly increased in chronic wounds, leading to breakdown of the ECM and either delayed, or failure of, re-epitheliasation. Finally, keratinocytes fail to migrate in chronic wounds due to high levels of inhibitory cytokines, elevated protease levels, and faulty ECM deposition.

Key points

* Acute wounds do not follow the same sequence of healing as chronic wounds which get 'stuck' in the inflammatory and proliferative stages of healing.
* Local and systemic factors and concomitant diseases can delay healing in both acute and chronic wounds.
* Chronic wounds contain cells that are unresponsive to the growth factor signals needed for wound repair.
* As the population ages, surgical and traumatic wounds will become more prevalent in older people, and will be slow to heal.

Pressure ulcers

A pressure ulcer is 'an area of localised damage to the skin and underlying tissue caused by pressure, shear, friction and/or a combination of these' (European Pressure Ulcer Advisory Panel [EPUAP], 1999) (_Figure 1.1_). They occur in all types of patients, including those traditionally thought to be 'not at risk', such as children and maternity patients. Despite the fact that it is believed that up to 95% of pressure ulcers are preventable, the prevalence remains high with a recent audit across five European countries suggesting that almost one in five hospital inpatients (18.1%) may have, or develop, a pressure ulcer (EPUAP, 2002a). The costs associated with both prevention and management of pressure ulcers are high. A recent estimate suggested that their cost in the UK was between £1.4 and £2.1 billion annually (approximately 4% of the NHS total spend) (Bennett _et al_, 2004).

They develop in patients who have one or more predisposing factors, often described as risk factors. These risk factors may be categorised as extrinsic (external) or intrinsic (internal).

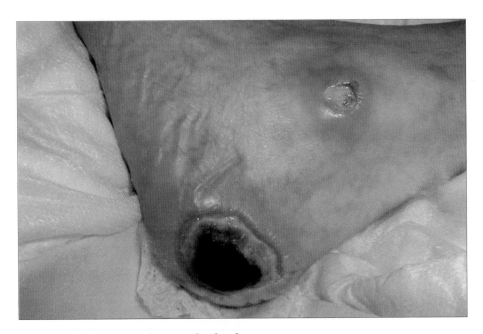

Figure 1.1: Pressure ulcer to the heel

Extrinsic factors

Extrinsic factors are the direct application of pressure shearing forces and, to a lesser extent, friction. Some texts also describe the presence of moisture on the skin as an external factor.

Any individual is able to withstand the application of even high amounts of pressure to the body for a short period of time. However, over time, the external pressure affects the underlying tissue. As the tissues are compressed the blood supply becomes compromised. If the individual moves and relieves the pressure, the blood supply is restored and damage does not occur. If the pressure is unrelieved, it will eventually lead to an area of oxygen and nutritional depletion with localised cell and tissue death. The pressure is much higher over boney prominences as the tissues are compressed between two hard surfaces, hence the fact that the majority of pressure ulcers occur over a boney prominence.

Shear is an internal force which causes the internal tissues and vasculature to be twisted and stretched – this may eventually result in tearing of the vessels causing further local damage. The narrowing and stretching of the blood vessels also means that it is easier to occlude them by applying external pressure; therefore, the element of shear increases the tissue's susceptibility to external pressure. Friction is a superficial force causing damage to the surface of the skin. The presence of moisture on the skin, whether due to incontinence, sweating, or wound exudate, causes over-hydration of the skin, increasing its susceptibility to damage. It has been suggested that these moisture lesions differ from pressure ulcers as they occur due to chemical irritation or maceration in the sacral or ischial areas, but do not involve bony prominences (Defloor and Schoonhoven, 2004).

Intrinsic factors

Intrinsic factors are numerous and varied and relate to the body's ability to mount a response to the external factors (*Table 1.1*).

Risk assessment tools are considered essential in the identification and prevention of pressure ulcers in individuals at risk. All risk assessment tools consider the extrinsic and intrinsic factors which may predispose an individual to pressure ulcer development, and suggest that interventions should be directed to those most vulnerable.

The most frequently used risk assessment tools are Waterlow (1985), Norton (1962), and Braden (1989; 2005).

Table 1.1: Intrinsic risk factors	
Immobility	The normal response to pressure is to move patients who are immobile, or who are less able or unable to move, and so endure the pressure for far longer time periods
Respiratory disease	The blood supply carries less oxygen, therefore hypoxia and tissue death occur more quickly
Circulatory disorders	Where the blood supply is compromised, it is easier for pressure to completely occlude the vessel
Poor nutrition	Poor nutrition is associated with being underweight, or conversely, obesity — both increase the risk of pressure damage. Also, a balanced diet is required for tissue repair
Age	In premature babies and young children, the skin is not mature and there are also differences in the weight distribution, for example, premature/new babies have larger, heavier heads (in relation to their overall body) than adults. Older adults have changes in the skin which result in reduction in elasticity and resilience. Additionally, increasing age is associated with occurrence of multiple disease pathologies which may impact on the risk status

Pressure ulcer grading differs from risk assessment, as it assesses and determines the predominant type of tissue affected, such as the dermis and epidermis (EPUAP, 2002b). Grading pressure ulcers should not be used to monitor the pressure ulcer's wound healing progress, as they do not progress from one grade to the next (Defloor and Schoonhoven, 2004). The early identification of pressure ulcers from other lesions allows preventative measures to be taken, and makes it possible to limit the severity of the pressure ulcer as far as possible.

Key points

❖ Pressure ulcers affect patients of all ages and types.
❖ The prevention and management of pressure ulcers is expensive in both financial and personal cost to the patient.
❖ The majority of pressure ulcers are preventable.
❖ Risk assessment and implementation of an appropriate treatment plan are essential.

Leg ulcers

Leg ulceration is a common chronic disease, with the prevalence of patients receiving care from healthcare professionals being estimated at approximately 0.11–0.18%. The percentage of people suffering from leg ulcer recurrence is likely to be 1–2% (Briggs and Closs, 2003). The financial costs of caring for these patients is high, with costs estimated to be in the region of £400 million (Bosanquet, 1992). Treatment of patients with leg ulceration can be complex, expensive and not always effective (Dunn, 1998). Although perceived as primarily a disease of the elderly, many patients' (25% of women and 45% of men) first episode of ulceration occurs before the age of sixty, and for 40% of those who are still working, the ulcer has an impact on their earning capacity (Callam *et al*, 1988).

In addition, the costs to the patient in terms of reduced quality of life, pain, and suffering are becoming more widely recognised (Anderson, 2000; Charles, 2004; Franks *et al*, 2003). Leg ulceration is a disease which, even with appropriate management, frequently recurs and single episodes of ulceration may last for many years. It is not surprising that patients describe living with a leg ulcer as a 'forever healing process' (Chase *et al*, 1997).

Leg ulcers occur for many reasons, but the most frequently described causes are: venous disease, arterial disease, and a mixture of arterial and venous disease (Maloney and Grace, 2004). In a systematic review of the literature, Briggs and Closs (2003) identify that the frequency with which these reasons are identified as the predominant cause of ulceration varies considerably between studies. This reflects the lack of agreed definitions for the underlying diseases, and considerable variation around what wounds have been included in the studies, for example, some studies include pressure ulcers to the heel and diabetic foot ulcers, while others exclude them. These inclusions and exclusions would have an impact on the percentages of other disease processes present. However, in a summary table, Briggs and Closs (2003) suggest that 37–81% are attributable to venous disease, 9–22% to arterial disease, and 7.1–26% to mixed venous/arterial disease.

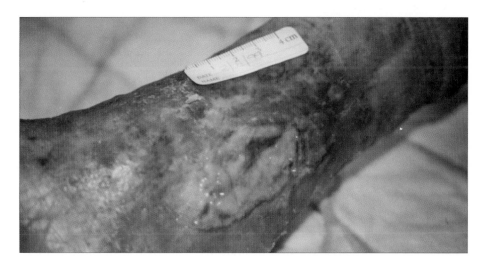

Figure 1.2: Venous leg ulcer

As leg ulcers are primarily a symptom of an underlying disease process, their management relies (where possible) on correction of the problem, following full assessment through Doppler, Duplex scan or pulse oximetry. This may include correction of underlying venous disease using compression therapy or surgery to restore arterial function. For patients, the main objectives are frequently related to symptom management, controlling exudate, reducing pain, and preventing cross-infection. As leg ulcers can take some considerable time to heal, engaging the patient in the process of care is imperative.

Clinical guidelines that identify assessment and management pathways for patients with leg ulceration are widely available (Royal College of Nursing Institute [RCNI], 1998; Scottish Intercollegiate Guidelines Network [SIGN] 1998), and many localities now offer specialist leg ulcer services which may be either nurse-led, or multidisciplinary, 'one stop' type services, that include access to dermatology and/or vascular services.

> **Key points**
>
> ❖ Leg ulcers frequently occur before the age of sixty.
> ❖ Identifying the underlying aetiology is crucial in determining an appropriate management plan.
> ❖ Patients frequently experience pain and other unwelcome symptoms which should be identified within the objectives of care.

Diabetic foot ulcers

Foot complications are common among people with diabetes. Approximately 20–40% will have neuropathy (the figure varies depending upon how this is defined and measured), and approximately 5% have a foot ulcer (MacIntosh *et al*, 2003). Although frequently referred to as one aetiology, 'the diabetic foot' is a group of syndromes, including the neuropathies (sensory, motor and autonomic), ischaemia and infection, which either singularly, or in combination, lead to the development of foot ulceration.

Neuropathy

Neuropathy affects the nervous system and it is this effect that impairs the individual's ability to mount a normal physiological response.

Sensory neuropathy affects the systems that transmit the signal of pain or sensation. Small fibre neuropathy affects the pain and temperature perception; large fibre neuropathy affects proprioception. Patients with sensory neuropathy may have completely insensate feet, which can cause them to sustain injuries from mechanical, thermal or chemical trauma, without being aware of having done so. The injury may go undiscovered for some time until other symptoms, such as bleeding, infection, or malodour, alert the individual. Sensory neuropathy may also present as increased or altered sensation, with some patients having hypersensitivity to touch. Usually, neuropathy is associated with poor glycaemic control, but starting insulin therapy can also precipitate a painful insulin neuritis.

Autonomic neuropathy affects the ability to sweat: sweating bathes the feet in sebum and keeps the skin well-hydrated. It also provides a bacterial barrier to invading microorganisms. When this function is reduced or lost, the skin becomes dry and cracks easily. Deep fissures can form which are prone to bacterial or fungal growth.

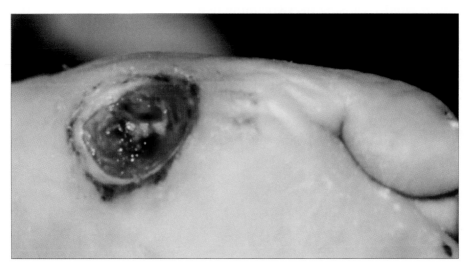

Figure 1.3: Diabetic foot ulcer

Motor neuropathy affects the small muscles of the foot leading to atrophy which, in turn, leads to collapse of the joints and the creation of abnormal pressure points as the weight-bearing load is distributed onto other parts of the foot. This abnormal weight distribution initiates a protective response to pressure, ie. the build up of callous in the area. When large amounts of hard callous form this, in itself, can act as a focal point for pressure causing underlying pressure damage.

Ischaemia

Poor circulation related to peripheral vascular disease (PVD) results in a reduced blood supply to the foot and lower leg — approximately 50% of foot pulses are absent in diabetic patients. While ischaemia alone is rarely the cause of ulceration, it is frequently implicated in delayed healing and increased risk of infection.

Infection

The metabolic abnormalities associated with diabetes, for example, impaired migration of neutrophils and macrophages, seem to predispose the wounds to infection (Falanga, 2000). Polymicrobial infection may spread rapidly, causing overwhelming tissue destruction. Absence of the protective pain function means that the initial signs of infection may not be noticed, and, all diabetic patients with wounds should be regularly and carefully assessed for the presence of infection, the major reason for amputation in diabetic feet (MacIntosh *et al*, 2003).

Key points

❖ Diabetic foot ulceration is a major cause of limb amputation.
❖ Ulceration usually occurs because of a combination of problems.
❖ Loss of protective pain sensation increases the risk of sustaining trauma.
❖ Development of infection in a diabetic foot ulcer may be limb- or life-threatening.

Burns

Minor burns and scalds are one of the most common reasons why patients attend A & E departments (approximately 150,000 new patients per year, Wardrope and Edhouse, 1999). Generally, adults with more than 15% burns or children with more than 10% burns are treated in specialised burn units (Dealey, 2005). Although they are all caused by excessive heat, the cause of burns can be broken down into four main categories: thermal, chemical, electrical and radiation.

❖ Thermal damage may be wet or dry (for example, a scald — wet, or a flame burn — dry).
❖ Chemical damage is caused by contact with caustic substances, either acid or alkaline. Damage to vital organs may occur if the substances pass into the blood stream. It is important to determine the causative agent as this may affect the subsequent management.

❖ Electrical burns occur when a current is passed through the body. These burns often appear less severe externally, with the majority of the damage being internal.
❖ Radiation damage occurs from planned or accidental exposure to radiotherapy (including sunlight).

Carrougher (1998) suggests that the type of burn injury is often age-related (_Table 1.2_).

Table 1.2: Most common burn injuries by age group	
Age group	**Common burn injuries**
0–4 years	Scalds (spill or bath-related) Residential fires Household chemicals (topical or ingested) Household electrical injuries (electrical cord bites)
5–14 years	Residential fires Risk-taking behaviour (fireworks, fire setting)
15–24 years	Automobile associated Work-related
25–64 years	Work-related
>65 years	Scalds Careless smoking, cooking accidents

Source: Carrougher, 1998

Burns vary in their depth and severity and this may be used to classify the extent of the damage.

❖ _Superficial burns:_ damage purely the epidermis and, for this reason, they may be extremely painful.
❖ _Superficial partial-thickness burns:_ involve the epidermis and the outermost layers of the dermis. They present as blisters and oedema.
❖ _Deep partial-thickness burns:_ penetrate and damage the deeper layers of the dermis. They often present as white areas with blisters.
❖ _Full-thickness burns:_ travel completely through the skin into the subcutaneous tissues and may affect deeper structures, such as muscle or bone. They appear as hard white, cherry red, or grey leathery tissue and are usually insensate.

Whatever the cause of the injury, the damage occurs in three dimensions which may be described as areas or zones of injury. The central zone of coagulation is the focus of the damage. In full-thickness burns it will appear white, leathery and insensate, and will not repair without significant scar formation. In partial-thickness burns, this area will be red, blistered and very painful. The second zone immediately surrounding this is the zone of stasis; in this area the cells are damaged but not destroyed. Oedema may form causing ischaemia and extension of the zone of coagulation. The outer area of the burn is the zone of hyperaemia, an area of minor cell damage but with increased blood flow as it supplies the necessary oxygen and nutrients to the more damaged areas.

After burn injury, oedema forms rapidly reaching a maximum at approximately twelve to twenty-four hours post injury. This can impair the delivery of oxygen and nutrients to the local area and increase the susceptibility to infection. The reasons for oedema formation are extremely complicated, but it is as a result of local and systemic inflammatory mediators which initiate the healing process and signal for other cells and mediators to arrive at the area.

Key points

* There are four main types of burns.
* Identification of the underlying cause is essential as it may affect management.
* Many burn injuries are preventable.
* Many burn injuries require specialist care and management.

Surgical wounds

Surgical wounds involve minimal tissue damage and are usually clean and sited anatomically to avoid major blood vessels and nerves. The acute, elective surgical wound in a patient with a healthy immune system provides optimal conditions for wound healing. However, not all surgical wounds heal without complications, and they may occur as a result of poor surgical technique, or significant trauma.

The majority of surgical wounds can be closed within six to twelve hours, provided that they are not contaminated. Bacterial contamination of surgical wounds is usually minimal but can be severe in dirty conditions, such as faecal peritonitis. Surgical wounds can be classified as clean, clean-contaminated, contaminated, and dirty. Surgical wounds are allowed to heal either by primary, secondary or tertiary intention (_Table 1.3_).

Table 1.3: Types of healing in surgical wounds	
Primary intention	Wound edges are approximated and closed at the time of surgery
Secondary intention	Wound is left open following surgery, and allowed to heal by the combined processes of granulation, contraction and epithelialisation
Tertiary intention (delayed primary closure)	Wound is left open following surgery for a short time. The wound edges are then carefully approximated and the wound closed

There are many factors affecting the healing of acute surgical wounds. Intrinsic factors, ie. those that influence the individual systemically, include:

- concurrent conditions
- age
- nutritional status
- dehydration
- psychological state
- medication and tissue perfusion.

Wounds healing by secondary or tertiary intention may not follow the regulated process of acute wound healing. This type of acute surgical wound that heals slowly or fails to heal can be considered to be chronic.

The patient's physical environment before, during, and after surgery, are examples of extrinsic factors affecting healing of surgical incisions. Surgical technique and wound closure techniques will also affect healing. Wound infection is the major cause of delayed healing, or non-healing, in surgical wounds. A large epidemiological study has shown that risk of surgical wound infection was increased by smoking, higher body mass index (BMI), haematoma formation, malignancy, increased numbers of people in theatre, use of adherent dressings, and skin closure times >10 days (Reilly, 2002). This study demonstrates how small changes in post-operative wound care can have a positive impact on patient outcomes.

The length of time a patient spends in hospital before surgery has been shown to increase the risk of surgical wound infection. Preoperative skin preparation also influences the risk of infection. Using electric razors or hair clippers, or leaving the operation site unshaved, has been linked to lower rates of infection, than use of non-electric razors to remove hair (Cruse and Foord, 1980). During the intraoperative period, the type of surgical procedure influences the risk of infection, and surgical procedures are

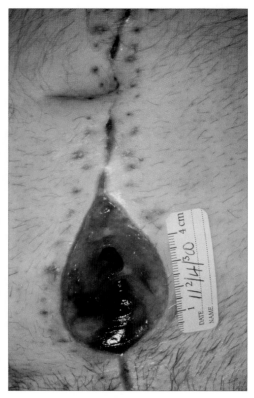

Figure 1.4: Dehisced surgical wound (abdominal)

classified depending on their risk of infection. Longer operations significantly increase the risk of infection, one study determined that the infection rate doubled for each hour the surgery proceeded (Cruse and Foord, 1980). Good surgical technique, in which the surgeon handles the tissues carefully, removes devitalised tissue, ensures adequate wound drainage and closes the wound by carefully approximating the wound edges, thereby minimising dead space, and achieves closure without putting excessive tension on the tissues, helps to reduce the risk of infection.

Management of the stress response in the immediate post-operative period is vital as the release of catecholamines into the circulation causes vasoconstriction, leading to hypoxia, hypovolaemia, hypothermia and pain. Poor tissue perfusion is associated with an increased risk of surgical wound infection.

Key points

❖ Wound infection is a key outcome indicator of surgery.
❖ Evidence-based practice can reduce the risk of surgical wound infection.
❖ Wound dressings for surgical wounds should be low-adherent.
❖ Wound closure materials should be removed within ten days.

Traumatic wounds

There are many types of traumatic wounds ranging from minor abrasions to extensive, life-threatening injuries (*Table 1.4*). A traumatic wound occurs when the body is subjected to a force that exceeds the strength of the skin or underlying tissues (Whiteside and Moorehead, 1999). Traumatic wounds can be classified as tidy or untidy. A tidy wound generally has a clean incision, is uncontaminated, is less than six hours old, and is caused by low-energy trauma. In contrast, an untidy wound has an irregular, ragged edge, is more than twelve hours old, is contaminated, and usually caused by high-energy trauma.

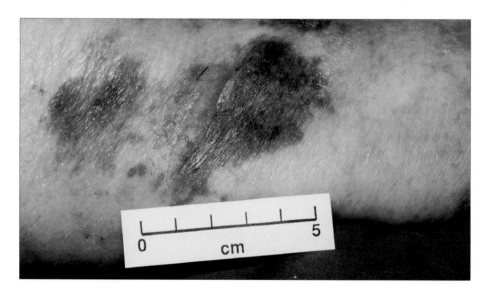

Figure 1.5: Traumatic wound — skin tear on arm

Table 1.4: Types of traumatic wounds and their causes

Skin tears/flaps	These wounds occur as a result of an accidental knock or bump to friable skin. The epidermis is displaced but retains a blood supply. Re-application of the skin tear/flap to the wound edges can facilitate healing
Grazes/ abrasions	These are superficial injuries where the skin is rubbed or torn, usually as a result of a fall. Wounds should be thoroughly cleansed to remove debris as a result of the injury
Lacerations	These are wounds caused by blunt trauma, which has split or torn the skin, forming jagged wound edges. Thorough wound assessment should be carried out to rule out the involvement of any underlying structure trauma
Penetration/ stab wounds	Knives, bullets or other sharp missiles are responsible for these wounds. Entry wounds may be small but investigation should determine if underlying structures are involved

Most major traumatic wounds are not life-threatening unless accompanied by serious haemorrhage. The first priority of treatment is, therefore, resuscitation, followed by assessment of the injury. It is important to determine how the injury occurred, as the extent of the force causing the tissue damage will determine the characteristics of the injury and subsequent management. Thorough examination of the patient is required to identify all injuries as this may not be immediately apparent.

To achieve a successful outcome, traumatic wounds should be managed using the principles described in *Table 1.5* (Rosen and Cleary, 1991).

Key points

* The extent of the force determines the extent of injury.
* Traumatic wounds can be classified as tidy or untidy.
* The general principles of managing traumatic wounds focus on restoration of blood supply, debridement, exploration, wound irrigation, antibiotic and tetanus therapy.
* Closure of traumatic wounds should be made on an individual basis after all risk factors have been considered.

The decision to close a traumatic wound should be based on clinical judgement, as this type of wound is prone to invasive bacterial infection due to the presence of devitalised tissue, bacteria and foreign bodies. If in doubt, it is better to leave a traumatic wound open to allow healing by secondary intention, or to close it at a later date by delayed primary closure.

Table 1.5: Principles of traumatic wound management	
Blood supply	Adequate tissue perfusion is required to promote healing. Local contusion, fractures and penetrating injuries may sever or occlude major blood vessels. The competence of the circulation must be carefully assessed
Debridement	All necrotic and devitalised tissue must be promptly debrided from the wound to remove dirt and bacteria to minimise infection. Devitalised soft tissue will encourage bacterial growth and the anaerobic environment decreases leukocyte activity
Irrigation	Irrigation with normal saline is required to remove haematomas and contaminants, such as dirt and road grease, to reduce the risk of infection. Care must be taken to avoid causing additional tissue trauma and oedema which decreases host defences
Exploration	Thorough exploration of traumatic wounds is required to identify damage to deep structures which should be performed under local or general anaesthetic. Blood vessel, nerve and tendon injuries are then repaired, as appropriate, to restore function
Antibiotics	Antibiotic prophylaxis should be administered as appropriate. Antibiotic therapy should never replace adequate wound irrigation and debridement. Prophylaxis is advisable when the wound is heavily contaminated, or, the patient's resistance is compromised
Tetanus	Tetanus caused by *Clostridium tetani* requires an anaerobic environment which can be minimised by thorough surgical debridement. If necessary, a booster dose of tetanus toxin can be administered

Conclusion

The relatively recent development of tissue viability as a speciality has focused on improving healing rates of patients with a wide range of wounds. It is now realistic to expect that, with evidence-based care, most wounds will heal uneventfully within a reasonable time-frame. Despite overall improvements in care, a small but significant proportion of wounds fail to heal and have a major impact on the patient's quality of life.

Although health professionals appreciate that many inter-related factors impair wound healing, these are not always easily identified in clinical practice. This book emphasises the importance of linking clinical observation skills to the underlying wound pathophysiology, so that abnormal changes are quickly identified, and appropriate therapeutic action implemented. It is now possible to collect a wide range of information during on-going wound assessment to facilitate clinical decision-making and to help identify when therapeutic interventions should be introduced, or modified, to accelerate healing.

The principles of evidence-based wound management centre around the importance of removing the underlying causes of the wound, optimising the local wound environment and preventing further tissue breakdown. The wound should also be considered within the wider patient context, ensuring that health professionals consider ways of maximising patient and carer involvement and, in some cases, the need for long-term support.

References

Agren MS, Steenfos H H, Dabelsteen S *et al* (1999) Proliferation and mitogenic response to PDGF-BB of fibroblasts isolated from chronic venous leg ulcers is ulcer-age dependent. *J Invest Dermatol* **112**(4): 463–9

Anderson I (2000) Quality of life and leg ulcer patients: will NHS reform address patient need? *Br J Nurs* **9**(13): 830–40

Bates-Jensen B, Wethe J (1998) Acute surgical wound management. In: Sussman C, Bates-Jensen B, eds. *Wound Care: A Collaborative Practice Manual for Physical Therapists and Nurses*. Aspen, Maryland: 219–30

Bennett G, Dealey C, Posnett J (2004) The cost of pressure ulcers in the UK. *Age Ageing* **33**: 230–5

Bosanquet N (1992) Costs of venous ulcers: From maintenance therapy to investment programmes. *Phlebology* **1**(Suppl): 44–6

Boxter E, Maynard C (1999) The management of chronic wounds: factors that affect nurses' decision-making. *J Wound Care* **8**(8): 409–12

Braden BJ, Bergstrom N (1989) Clinical utility of the Braden scale for predicting pressure sore risk. *Decubitus* **2**(3): 44–51

Braden BJ, Maklebust J (2005) Preventing pressure ulcers with the Braden scale: an update on this easy to use tool. *Am J Nurs* **105**(6): 70–2

Briggs M, Closs SJ (2003) The prevalence of leg ulceration: a review of the literature. *EWMA J* **3**(2): 14–20

Callam MJ, Harper DR, Dale JJ, Ruckley CV (1988) Chronic leg ulceration: socio-economic aspects. *Scott Med J* **33**: 358–60

Carrougher G (1998) *Burn Care and Therapy*. Mosby, St Louis

Charles H (2004) Does leg ulcer treatment improve patients' quality of life? *J Wound Care* **13**(6): 209–13

Chase S, Melloni M and Savage A (1997) A forever healing process: The lived experience of venous ulcer disease. *J Vasc Nurs* **10**(2): 73–8

Chen WY, Abatangelo G (1999) Functions of hyaluronan in wound repair. *Wound Rep Regen* **7**: 79–89

Cruse PJE, Foord R (1980) The epidemiology of wound infection. A 10-year prospective study of 62 939 wounds. *Surg Clin North Am* **60**(1): 27–40

Dealey C (2005) *The Care of Wounds*. 3rd edn. Blackwell Science Ltd, Oxford

Defloor T, Schoonhoven L (2004) Inter-rater reliability of the EPUAP pressure ulcer classification system using photographs. *J Clin Nurs* **13**(8): 952–9

Dunn C (1998) Clinically effective leg ulcer care. *Nurs Times* **94**: 47

European Pressure Ulcer Advisory Panel (1999) *Pressure Ulcer Treatment Guidelines*. EPUAP, Oxford

European Pressure Ulcer Advisory Panel (2002a) Summary report on the prevalence of pressure ulcers. *EPUAP Rev* **4**(2)

European Pressure Ulcer Advisory Panel (2002b) Guide to pressure ulcer grading. *EPUAP Rev* **3**: 75

Falanga V, ed (2000) *Text Atlas of Wound Management*. Martin Dunitz, London

Flanagan M (1998) The impact of change on the tissue viability nurse specialist: 1. *Br J Nurs* **7**(11): 648–57

Franks PJ, McCulloch L, Moffat CJ (2003) Assessing quality of life in patients with chronic leg ulceration using the Medical Outcomes Short Form — 36 questionnaire. *Ostomy Wound Management* **49**(2): 26–37

JeffcoateWJ, Harding KG (2003) Diabetic foot ulcers. *Lancet* **361**: 1545–51

Lucker KA, Kenrick M (1995) Towards knowledge-based practice: an evaluation of a method of dissemination. *Int J Nurs Stud* **32**(1): 59–67

MacIntosh A, Peters J, Young R, Hutchinson A, Chiverton R, Clarkson S *et al* (2003) *Prevention and Management of Foot Problems in Type 2 Diabetes: Clinical Guideline and Evidence*. University of Sheffield, Sheffield

Maloney M, Grace P (2004) Understanding the underlying causes of chronic leg ulceration. *J Wound Care* **13**(6): 215–18

Norton D, McLaren R, Exton-Smith AN (1962) *An investigation of geriatric nursing problems in hospital*. National Corporation for the Care of Old People, London

Price P, Enoch S (2004) Cellular, molecular and biochemical differences in the pathophysiology of healing between acute wounds, chronic wounds and wounds in the aged. Available online at: http://worldwidewounds.com

Reilly J (2002) Evidence-based surgical wound care on surgical wound infection. *Br J Nurs* (supplement) **11**(16): S4–S12

Royal College of Nursing Institute (1998) *Clinical Practice Guidelines. The Management of Patients with Venous Leg Ulcers*. RCN Institute, York/Manchester

Rosen J, Cleary J (1991) Surgical management of wounds. *Clin Podiatr Med Surg* **8**(4): 891–907

Schultz GS, Sibbald RG, Falanga V, Ayello EA, Dowsett C *et al* (2003) Wound bed preparation: a systematic approach to wound management. *Wound Rep Regen* **1**(2) supplement: S1–S28

Scottish Intercollegiate Guidelines Network (1998) *The Care of Patients with Chronic Leg Ulcers: A National Clinical Guideline*. SIGN, Edinburgh

Wardrope J, Edhouse JA (1999) *The Management of Wounds and Burns*. Oxford University Press, Oxford

Waterlow J (1985) Pressure sores: a risk assessment card. *Nurs Times* **81**(48): 49–55

Whiteside M, Moorehead R (1999) Traumatic Wounds: principles of management. In: Miller M, Glover D, eds. *Wound Management: theory and practice*. NT Books, Emap, Oxford: 37–45

Chapter 2

Progression to healing

Martyn Butcher

As clinicians, we are faced with the dilemma of how best we can facilitate the progression of our patient's wound through the healing process to a successful outcome; namely, the production of a healed wound where tissue integrity is restored. Successful management of the wound relies on the clinician's ability to assess structures and tissues involved, recognition of delaying factors and the desired outcomes, and understanding of how interventions (dressings or therapies) can modify the healing process to produce an enhanced effect.

The use of a model (for example, the Wound Progression Model, *Figure 2.1*) can help the clinician identify the expected logical progression of the wound from one wound state to the next.

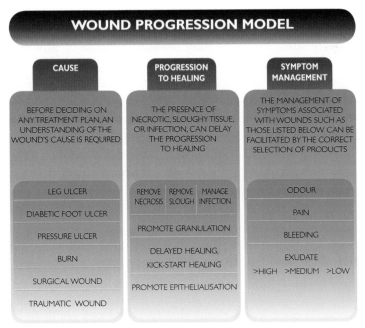

Figure 2.1: The Wound Progression Model

The Wound Healing Continuum (*Figure 2.2*) (Gray *et al*, 2005) also provides a logical basis, not only for wound classification by visual assessment, but also for guiding the clinician towards matching assessment with expected outcomes. In this way, it can help in alerting when interventions are not achieving their desired goals.

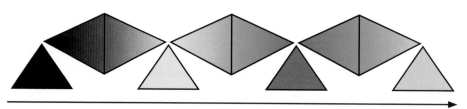

Necrotic, necrotic/sloughy, sloughy, sloughy/granulating, granulating/epithelialisation and epithelialisation

Figure 2.2: The Wound Healing Continuum (Gray *et al*, 2005)

The system builds on the simplistic black, yellow, red, pink (necrotic, sloughy, granulating, epithelialising) colour classification devised by Cuzzell (1988), and later expanded and developed by Krasner (1995), to include more subtle changes that occur between these clear boundaries. Wounds are classified as black, black to yellow, yellow, yellow to red, red, red to pink, and pink. The aim is to move the wound from left to right (black to pink) along the continuum, through the various stages until closure occurs. Wounds may initially present at any point along the line, however, under normal circumstances, successful progression should always be towards the right of the continuum. Wounds that revert to a previous status or which appear to decline (move left along the continuum), should be seen as a deterioration requiring further investigation or alterations in intervention.

The following sections are designed to aid the clinician in recognising the basic tissue types and provide some advice on appropriate treatment strategies to progress the wound to healing.

Necrotic tissue

Necrotic tissue is once living tissue that has died as a result of ischaemia. This may be precipitated by arterial or capillary occlusion (as in the case of pressure damage or in peripheral vascular disease), vascular insufficiency following surgery, damage from chemicals and excessive heat, and infection (O'Brien, 2003). The appearance of necrotic tissue is dependent on its water content and the degree of mummification that has occurred. Newly ischaemic tissue will be similar in texture to normal tissue, but will have a purple hue. In time, this tissue will dehydrate and become hard and leathery. At this time, it may be referred to as eschar. This dried tissue is inflexible and may eventually become rigid.

If this dead tissue is exposed to moisture, this desiccating process can be reversed and the ischaemic tissue will soften and become brown, yellow or grey. If left in place, putrefaction continues as a result of bacterial growth and the action of the individual's own immune system.

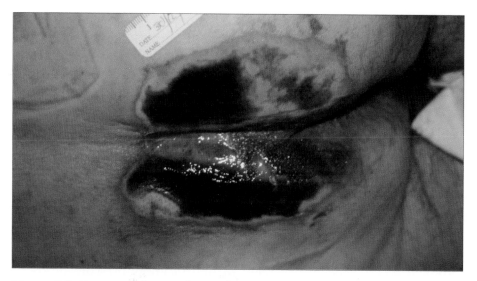

Figure 2.3: Pressure ulcer with necrotic tissue

Why remove dead tissue?

The presence of necrotic tissue in the wound can a have a number of negative effects on the healing process. By acting as a covering to the wound bed, it effectively prevents the assessment of the underlying structures (Vowden and Vowden, 1999). This can have serious consequences, particularly in the management of acute trauma when decisions on future wound management may be determined by the severity of the wound and structures involved. The presence of devitalised protein in the wound provides an ideal nutrient to pathological bacteria, enabling them to multiply to harmful levels and can, therefore, act as a pool for infection. Gram-negative and anaerobic organisms can lead to foul smelling odours, increasing social isolation. The presence of necrotic material in the wound also enhances the inflammatory phase of healing and can lead to the production of excessive inflammatory cytokines which, in turn, damage regenerating collagen fibres and growth factors (Leaper, 2002).

When should the clinician leave necrotic material *in situ*?

Generally, the presence of necrotic tissue is seen as a delaying factor in wound healing, however, there are exceptions to this paradigm. In the absence of adequate vascular supply, tissue regeneration can be inhibited or, indeed, absent. Removal of necrotic tissue will expose underlying structures to the effects of desiccation and bacterial ingress. This can lead to further tissue death and wound extension. In certain circumstances, the clinician should leave necrotic tissue *in situ* and aim to improve dehydration. This reduces the possibility of bacterial growth and can lead to successful auto-amputation of the area. Dry or iodine-based antimicrobial dressings can be helpful in this process. One particular example of the benefits of 'active non-intervention' is found in the patient with peripheral vascular disease who develops dry ischaemic necrosis of the toes. In this case, attempts to rehydrate the eschar leads to moist necrosis that can have disastrous consequences if the wound becomes infected (Hampton, 1997). Other instances where this approach may be indicated include the management of full-thickness pressure ulcers in the terminally ill. If a necrotic cap covers the wound but does not cause distress to the patient, it may be preferable to leave this *in situ* if palliation, rather than wound healing, is the desired outcome (Leaper, 2002).

In most cases, the aim of treatment should be the removal of dead tissue. The process of debridement (the removal of devitalised tissue) can be achieved in a number of ways.

Autolytic debridement

In most cases, if kept moist, dead material will naturally degrade. This process is mediated by leukocytes and, in some cases, the bacterial load within the wound. Matrix metalloproteinases (enzymes released by white blood cells as part of the natural inflammatory response) break down protein bonds and lead to the sloughing away of non-viable tissue (Thomas *et al*, 1999; Baharestani, 1999). Interventions aimed at enhancing autolysis involve maintenance of a moist or saturated environment. Products, such as hydrocolloids and semi-permeable films, trap fluid in the wound bed and can lead to rehydration. Hydrogels can be particularly effective as they donate additional moisture, providing a wet wound bed. However, care must be taken to prevent surrounding tissue from becoming macerated, and the time taken for debridement to occur may be protracted (Leaper, 2002).

The recent availability of commercial honey preparations has made them an alternative to hydrogels. Honey-based ointments (predominantly Manuka honey), are applied to the necrotic tissue and covered with a semi-occlusive dressing. This rehydrates the eschar and draws fluid through the eschar by osmotic action. It is claimed that this process not only enhances the autolytic process, but also provides antimicrobial action against the overgrowth of pathogenic organisms (Molan, 2005).

Sharp debridement

The physical removal of dead tissue with sharp instruments, such as scissors or scalpel, is the fastest method of wound debridement. This should only be undertaken by appropriately trained, skilled, and competent practitioners (Vowden and Vowden, 1999). There needs to be a clear distinction made between surgical debridement and conservative sharp debridement (see *overleaf*).

Chemical debridement

Chemical debriding agents such as hydrogen peroxide and sodium hypochlorite (EUSOL) have been available for many years. While many of these have been proven to have bactericidal effects, research has shown that they can have toxic effects on healthy tissue and fibroblasts. In addition, they can cause pain on application. Their use is declining in regular wound care practice in the UK (Leaper, 2002).

Surgical debridement is usually undertaken in theatres and involves the removal of all non-viable and compromised tissue until a healthy bleeding wound bed is achieved. This is often undertaken as a one-step procedure. As live tissue will be disrupted in this process, anaesthetic (often general) is normally required.

Conservative sharp debridement is normally performed at the bedside. The skilled clinician trims or pares non-viable tissue away from viable tissue at, or above, the plain of viability. As live tissue is left intact, additional analgesia is not normally required. Conservative debridement may be undertaken in conjunction with other therapies, such as autolysis, to enhance healing rates (O'Brien, 2003), and may need to be undertaken serially until the wound bed is clear of debris.

Mechanical debridement

Necrotic tissue can be physically pulled from the wound bed. Traditionally, this has been achieved by the use of wet-to-dry dressings. Moist gauze is applied to the necrotic wound and the area covered by a non-occlusive, retaining bandage. The gauze dries out by evaporative loss over a number of hours. The dressing is subsequently removed, taking with it the adherent material. Despite the low cost of the dressings used, this method of wound debridement is not cost effective (Ovington, 2002). This form of therapy is rarely practiced in the UK now, due to the pain and trauma caused to the patient and wound bed, however, it is still practiced in some countries as the principle method of debridement.

More recent developments have led to the use of high-pressure irrigation and hydro-pool cleansing. Jets of warmed solution are used to loosen the bonds between the adherent necrotic material and the viable tissue. In many cases, these systems do seem to be clinically effective (Palmier and Trial, 2004), but require expensive equipment and have issues over equipment cleansing and cross-infection. The addition of ultrasound in pressure cleansing does improve results achieved but, unfortunately, increases cost considerably. This system tends to be reserved for specialist wound care centres.

Enzymatic debridement

Natural autolysis depends on the presence of both moisture and the appropriate enzymes to break down the firm proteinous bonds between the eschar and the wound bed. In the absence of the latter, synthetic and naturally occurring enzymes can be introduced to enhance the breakdown of non-viable tissue. Outside of the UK, North America and other parts of Europe, commercially available products are more frequently used. These enzymes include proteolytics, fibrinolytics and collaginases. It is recommended that these enzymes are applied often, once or twice daily, to a thoroughly cleansed wound bed and, to be effective, only used in the absence of silver products (Ayello _et al_, 2004). They are active in two ways. Firstly, by digesting the components of devitalised tissue (fibrin, cell debris and DNA, for example) and, secondly, by dissolving collagen that anchors this tissue to the wound bed (Ramundo and Wells, 2000). There is limited research and evidence in terms of randomised controlled trials to support the use of enzymes. However, clinical trials employing other methodologies have reported an increase in the speed of removal of devitalised tissue (Mosher _et al_, 1999).

Larval therapy

The ability of fly larvae to break down dead material has been recognised for many years. Recent developments in the breeding and sterilising of the larvae of the specific fly species, _Lucilia Sericata_, has enabled clinicians to induce deliberately a benign myasis in patients with necrotic wound burden. Larvae secrete potent proteolytic enzymes that break down necrotic material, producing a thick protein-rich broth on which they feed. In addition to breaking down dead tissues, the larvae are able to ingest and break down pathogenic organisms in the wound (Thomas _et al_, 1999). This can make their use in the infected or heavily colonised wound effective. While effective, larvae can be problematic to apply and, should their enzymes come in contact with healthy epidermis, this can cause excoriation (Thomas _et al_, 2003) similar to that seen in small bowel effluent contamination. However, this risk can be reduced by applying a hydrocolloid dressing around the wound margin. The clinician must also be aware of patient preference: not all patients or clinicians are happy dealing with larvae.

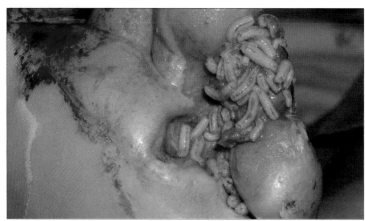

Figure 2.4: Larval therapy, reproduced by kind permission of ZooBiotic Ltd, Biosurgical Products

The choice of debridement method will depend on a number of factors, including the characteristics of the wound (infection, exudate, tissues involved and required rate of debridement), the patient's attitude, available skills and available resources (Vowden and Vowden, 2002)

Sloughy tissue

Wounds can be classified by the colour and nature of the tissue within their margins. Clinicians are often faced with wounds that appear yellow or grey in appearance. These are often referred to as 'sloughy' (Tong, 1999). However, it is important for the clinician to differentiate between the wound filled with slough and those with pus present (indicating possible infection), or those with viable pale tissue (such as adipose tissue) present.

Slough is generally soft, devitalised tissue that can build up on previously healthy material. Histologically, it does not have a defined structure, but is composed of fibrin, pus and significant volumes of proteinaceous material (Thomas, 2001). It may have a number of appearances from soft, sticky liquid to a more robust film. It may even appear as a stringy fibre-filled material. Once dried-out, it becomes yellow-brown and takes on a more fibrous or hardened appearance.

As with the necrotic wound, the presence of slough can slow the healing process by providing a foreign body reaction, prolonging the inflammatory stage and providing an environment that can act as a pool for infection. Generally, therefore, the clinician should aim to remove this tissue through the judicious use of appropriate debridement techniques (Tong, 1999).

As in the necrotic wound, rehydration with hydrocolloids, hydrogels or pre-moistened Hydrofiber® (ConvaTec) can be useful in preparing the wound for debridement (Vowden, 2004). Where slough is liquid, leakage of this fluid may result in strike-through of the dressing material or leakage onto surrounding skin. It may be necessary to manage this exudate with absorbent dressings. Alginates and Hydrofiber® are useful tools in the management of this fluid (Vowden, 2004).

Granulating tissue

New tissue is laid down in the wound by the action of fibroblasts. These cells are triggered into action by the presence of growth factors secreted by macrophages. The fibroblasts lay down fibrils of reticulum that are later converted to collagen. This process is highly dependent on energy and oxygen. New blood vessels grow through the clot matrix as a result of capillary budding (angiogenesis).

In healthy granulation, the tissue shows a bright red colouration and is bubbly in appearance due to the presence of new tissue and its highly vascular nature. This tissue is not covered with epithelium and so is prone to trauma and moisture loss.

Management of the granulating wound should provide an environment that is warm and moist and where structures are protected from trauma. These wounds can vary considerably in size, shape and exudate level. Dressing selection can, therefore, be problematic.

High to very highly exuding wounds

High levels of exudate can be caused by factors at three levels. Systemically, high exudate can be secondary to excessive fluid in the extracellular tissues. This fluid can drain out of the wound as a result of gravitational stasis. Conditions, such as cardiac oedema and ascites, may have a significant influence. Management of excessive exudate in these circumstances will require a multidisciplinary approach to disease management and may require systemic therapy. At a regional level, factors such as primary and secondary lymphoedema, venous hypertension, and postoperative oedema will need more localised management. Underlying function should be restored or enhanced wherever possible. This may require the use of external therapies, such as compression bandages, hosiery, intermittent compression therapy, or massage and manual lymphatic drainage. Local issues may include the presence of connecting fistulae, foreign bodies, acute and chronic inflammatory conditions and infection.

Deep, highly exuding wounds

Due to the highly vascular nature of granulation tissue and the large surface area afforded by deep wounds, high levels of exudate are not uncommon. The clinician's aim is to maintain tissue moisture without causing maceration of surrounding tissues. In addition, steps should be undertaken to promote further tissue growth without the formation of local dead-spaces, which would provide an environment for subsequent infection and abscess formation.

Traditionally, wounds such as these were packed with ribbon gauze soaked in a wide variety of solutions. Later techniques, using alginate (for example, Kaltostat™ [ConvaTec], Sorbsan™ [Unomedical], Seasorb soft™ [Coloplast]) and Hydrofiber® ribbons (for example, Aquacel™ [ConvaTec]), have proven more effective at encouraging new tissue growth and have been less traumatic for patients. Some specific cavity-filling foam dressings (for example, Allevyn™ Cavity [Smith and Nephew]) have proven to be an effective and time-efficient alternative (Berry *et al*, 1996).

Deep, lowly exuding wounds

If exudate levels fall, desiccation can quickly occur. This will slow or stop new tissue growth. In such scenarios, it is necessary to increase moisture levels. Amorphous hydrogels such as Granugel® (ConvaTec), Intrasite™ (Smith and Nephew), Purilon™ (Coloplast), Nu-Gel™ (Johnson and Johnson) and Aquaform™ (Unomedical) can all be of use. These need to be held in place with a secondary, semi-occlusive dressing and changed regularly to prevent them from drying out. Deep cavities may benefit from the properties of alginates/Hydrofiber® ribbons, which may be pre-moistened to prevent adherence and drying of the wound. Irrigation dressings, such as Tenderwet™ (Paul Hartmann), may help maintain moisture levels without the problems associated with gel leak and drip.

Shallow, highly exuding wounds

In shallow wounds, dressings should be chosen that can cope with exudate but which do not wick fluid onto the surrounding skin. Sheet alginate dressings are frequently used in combination with either a dressing pad or some other high absorbency secondary dressing. Hydrofiber® has many of the advantages of alginates and copes with additional fluid levels as it absorbs and retains. Sheet foam dressings have the ability to absorb exudate. Earlier versions acted like a simple bath sponge: while taking up fluid they were unable to lock this fluid away and so when pressure was applied to them (for instance, under compression bandages) they tended to leak. Later, more complex products are said to combine hydrophobic inner layers with hydrophilic cores and no-leak backing (for example, Allevyn™ [Smith and Nephew] and Biatain™ [Coloplast]). Some manufacturers now produce combination dressings. These may include multiple layers of various hydrophilic products. Some also include hydrophilic granulates similar to those found in disposable nappies and sanitary towels. This can greatly increase their absorbency.

Shallow, lowly exuding wounds

Foam dressings also have a part to play in this type of wound. By keeping a moist environment they prevent desiccation of delicate granulation tissue. More commonly used products include the hydrocolloids. These trap moisture as they gel and provide a low oxygen environment that further enhances angiogenesis.

Topical negative pressure (TNP) therapy

The development of topical negative pressure therapy (TNP) (VAC® Therapy™ [KCI Medical]) has resulted in a fundamental change in the management of many granulating wounds, particularly cavity wounds. The vacuum produced drains exudate away from the wound while maintaining a moist wound interface, and the semipermeable film drape maintains negative pressure but also acts as a highly efficient bacterial barrier. This can be of great assistance in managing the high exudate levels. Greatly enhanced localised angiogenesis, enhanced oxygen potential, and the stimulation of growth factors increases granulation tissue formation, while the dressing provides stability to the wound and reverse tissue expansion encourages wound contraction. In many scenarios, this should be considered the first treatment of choice. In some healthcare settings, funding and availability of this therapy can be problematic.

In the non-compromised individual, granulation occurs rapidly as the body fills the defect left by the initial trauma, however, in compromised individuals, granulation can be delayed. In such cases, the resultant tissue can appear pale in colour and look thin. Factors such as raised matrix metalloproteinase (MMP) levels, as seen in chronic wound fluid, can adversely affect tissue repair. New granulation tissue is broken down by these proteolytic enzymes as soon as they start to form. A number of products are now marketed at modulating these enzymes by either binding excessive numbers in their matrix (as in Hyalofill® [ConvaTec], Promogran™ [Johnson and Johnson] and Catrix™ [Valeant Pharmaceuticals]), or by modifying factors in the wound environment, such as pH and bacterial burden, so limiting their production (the claimed action of Cadesorb™ [Smith and Nephew] and a number of the silver-based compounds).

The presence of abnormally red, friable granulation may indicate the presence of high levels of bacteria in the wound (Gray *et al*, 2005; Stephen-Haynes, 2005). This phenomenon is often referred to as critical colonisation (Gray *et al*, 2005), indicating bacterial burden high enough to inhibit normal tissue regeneration, but without eliciting a host reaction. Management of this tissue needs to be targeted at reducing bacterial load to a point where the body's normal immune system can achieve a balance (see section on infection, *pp. 37–40*).

Overgranulation

Over-exuberant production of granulation tissue can pose a problem for the clinician. Such tissue is prone to damage and has a propensity to bleed. Once proud of surrounding epithelium, epidermal cover is difficult to establish. Overgranulation occurs as a result of prolonged inflammation, either from foreign material or the presence of high bacterial load. To date, there is little consensus on the best method of management for such wounds. Little research has been undertaken on the subject. There are two main reasons for this: the condition causes no discomfort or significant danger to the individual and so is not perceived as a major issue in research; and, secondly, due to the individual nature of these wounds and their relative scarcity, it is difficult to recruit sufficient number to achieve statistically significant outcomes.

Clinicians tend to use one or more of four options:

❖ *Antimicrobials:* due to the apparent link between bacterial numbers and the over-production of granulation tissue, many clinicians consider using topical antimicrobials, such as silver- or iodine-based products, as their first treatment option. These products are relatively easy to use and are accessible in most care settings.

❖ *Pressure:* granulation tissue frequently becomes oedematous in the presence of prolonged inflammation. Simple pressure on the tissue can reduce this and permit surrounding epidermal tissue to migrate over the wound surface. Such pressure can be applied with a foam dressing (adhesive foams are often used), or a hydrocolloid, both of which significantly reduce the height of the granulation tissue (Harris and Rolstad, 1994; Young, 1997). Alternatively, on the lower limb, the use of compression bandages may be of assistance.

❖ *Topical steroids:* topical gluco-corticosteroids are capable of reducing inflammation in underlying tissue. Many clinicians use potent steroids to reduce inflammation and induce shrinking of oedematous granulation. Although successful in many patients, it has to be remembered that topical steroid preparations, such as hydrocortisone cream 1%, are not licensed for this indication (Young, 1995). Corticosteroids can be easily absorbed by tissues. Prolonged use of these products can delay healing, prompt systemic absorption and lead to pigmentation changes. Therapy, therefore, has to be undertaken for a limited time-frame (seven days is normally adequate), and in small amounts (Dunford, 1999).

❖ **Caustic preparations:** it is possible to chemically burn back over granulation tissue. Invariably, this tissue is insensate and so pain relief is not normally required prior to the application of 95% silver nitrate to the moist tissue. This process is undertaken at subsequent dressings until the required effect is achieved. Special care needs to be taken not to touch the surrounding tissue, especially the delicate epithelial margins. If this does occur, delayed migration is likely. Due to the risk of damage to surrounding tissues, this treatment tends to be used as a final resort.

Delaying factors to granulation

There are a number of other factors that can also delay granulation. Wherever possible these need to be addressed to produce optimal healing conditions. External factors include: repeated trauma, pressure, desiccation, repeated cooling of tissues, the continued presence of foreign material and debris, chemical stressors, and smoking. Internal factors include: underlying disease processes that reduce circulation (eg. peripheral vascular disease, anaemia) and alter immune status, oxygen potential, and metabolic status. Age, body build and nutritional factors all have direct influences on the rate of granulation seen during the healing process.

Epithelial tissue

The aim of wound healing is to re-establish the continuity of tissue and to restore its normal function. In skin, this effectively means the covering of the wound bed with new epithelial tissue. The method by which this is achieved will depend on the particular features of the wound. In partial-thickness wounds, epidermal elements exist in the damaged tissues. Hair follicles and other skin structures, such as sweat glands, are lined with epidermal cells. These can multiply and migrate across the surface of the wound to produce a new epithelial layer, restoring skin integrity. This process is clearly seen in the healing of split-thickness skin graft donor sites. Here, epidermal cells can be seen to migrate out from each of the hair follicles until neighbouring areas of re-growth touch. When removing the dressings on partially-healed donor sites, the clinician will vividly see these small islands of epithelium as pink dots across the raw, granulating wound bed.

In full-thickness tissue loss, these epidermal structures are absent. Epidermal regeneration takes place by the gradual ingress of squamous epithelial tissue from the wound borders.

At the edge of all migrating epithelial tissue, the structures are delicate and the active edge is only one cell thick. For successful migration to take place it is essential that these cells are kept moist, warm and trauma-free. Desiccation of these tissues causes cell death and prevents further advancement. The clinician should ensure that the correct dressing material is employed to prevent damage and maintain a healing environment. There are a variety of products that can be successfully employed to modulate the environment.

Where exudate is low, a semi-permeable film will maintain moisture levels and protect tissues from desiccation and trauma. Hydrocolloid dressings and, where exudate is higher, sheet foams, provide a safe, warm environment for cell migration. It is essential to ensure that stripping of new epithelium does not occur. All products used must be non-adherent to the wound bed. Adhesive products can be particularly useful in that they minimise shearing forces between the dressing and the wound bed. This minimises friction that will disrupt cell migration. However, adhesive dressings need to be chosen with care to prevent damage to recently healed structures and prevent further damage to the peri-wound area. In addition, the clinician has to be aware that sensitivity to certain adhesives can occur among patients. Where this is known, alternative methods of fixation should be employed.

Skin grafts

Where the wound is large with significant areas of epidermal loss, it may be impractical to rely on re-epithelialisation from surrounding tissue. Due to the slow progress of this process, the wound bed will remain open for prolonged periods of time. This will increase the risk of subsequent infection and lead to the deposition of large amounts of scar tissue in the wound. This can result in extensive scarring which is not only unsightly, but can cause wound contracture reducing the efficiency of joints and underlying musculature.

In such cases, it may be more appropriate to apply new epidermal tissue to the surface of the wound, which can subsequently become integrated within the wound matrix and act as a reservoir for epidermal cells. This is the principle behind the use of skin grafts. Skin grafts are areas of skin (of varying thickness), harvested without a specific blood supply and then applied to an area denuded of epidermis. The graft is not attached to a new blood supply immediately, but rather it develops a new vascular supply from the underlying tissues. Skin grafts are classified according to their host donor relationship (Beldon, 2004).

Split skin grafts are made up of tissue that incorporates the epidermis with limited amounts of dermal elements. Full-thickness grafts contain both epidermis and dermis and will also carry skin structures such as hair follicles. Split skin grafts are used to cover large areas of epidermal loss (such as in the repair of major burns), but can have a poor cosmetic appearance and are generally not able to withstand high levels of wear and tear. Because of the amount of structures within them and their demands on nutrients such as oxygen, full-thickness grafts are limited in size. They have a lower graft to scar ratio, tend to contract less, and it is possible to predict their final colour. This, along with their improved texture and hair-bearing potential, makes them better suited in cosmetic and functional reconstructive surgery.

An **Autograft** is a piece of tissue removed from an individual and replaced on a different part of the same individual.

An **Allograft** is tissue removed from one individual and used on a different individual of the same species.

A **Xenograft** is tissue harvested from an individual and used on an animal of a different species (eg. pig skin used as a temporary skin substitute on humans).

Dressing choices in skin graft care are varied. The main focus of care should be to retain moisture in the newly applied graft to prevent desiccation and subsequent graft failure. Graft revascularisation can take up to ten days, during which time new capillary buds grow from the wound bed into the graft tissue. Lateral movement during this phase prevents the establishment of new circulation. The graft should be kept immobile. Collections of serous fluid or blood can be avoided by the use of gentle pressure to the graft but, if this occurs, it should be drained with a sterile needle or by carefully slitting the graft.

Whether healing of the wound is by tissue regeneration or tissue replacement with skin grafting, once full re-epithelialisation of the wound occurs, care is needed to protect delicate tissues from damage until such time as the tissue matures, and normal protective functions, such as sebaceous gland activity, are re-established and reasonable tensile strength is restored. This may require the use of protective dressings or emollient preparations for some time after closure. The length of time such measures take will depend on the extent of damage initially caused, the stresses the skin is likely to encounter, and the individual patient's constitution. This will need to be assessed on an individual patient basis.

Infected tissue

Whenever there is a break in the continuity of the skin there is the potential for bacterial ingress. The multiplication of bacteria in the wound robs natural tissues of vital nutrients and oxygen, and can cause the production of toxins that have a negative effect on healing. This can lead to local wound degradation and extension and generalised sepsis.

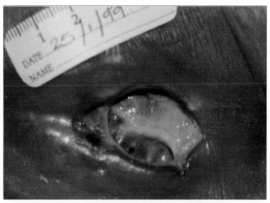

Figure 2.5: Infected pressure ulcer to sacrum

Early recognition of infection is essential if delays in wound healing are to be avoided. However, indicators such as wound swabs can be misleading as they can identify colonising bacteria as well as the causative organism, and provide us with retrospective data. More commonly, clinicians have to rely on clinical signs to provide the evidence of localised and spreading infection. Key signs may include:

- cellulitis and spreading erythema
- increasing odour and/or exudate
- abscess formation
- discoloration of the wound surface
- tissue breakdown.

More subtle changes, possibly indicating localised infection or bacterial overgrowth, may include:

- granulation tissue fragility
- increased pain and discomfort
- superficial pocketing or bridging
- a static, non-healing wound.

Gray *et al* (2005) describes wound colonisation and infection as a continuum (see *Figure 2.7*) that progresses from sterility, a transient condition seen in fresh thermal injuries, to systemic infection where the host defence mechanism is fully activated, and where signs of pathogenic activity may be seen some distance from the site of injury (eg. pyrexia, malaise). Treatment management needs to be tailored to the needs of the patient and their position along this continuum.

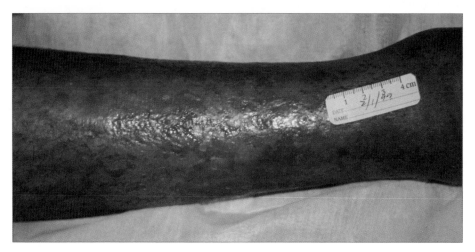

Figure 2.6: Cellulitis of the leg

Sterility

This is a short-lived status. Management should be aimed at minimising contamination of the wound with pathogenic organisms. Sterile, semi-occlusive dressings should be selected that are suitable for the structures involved, and which provide an environment where regeneration can take place.

Contamination

Bacteria are present in the wound, but are not reproducing or are at low levels. This is the normal state for most wounds at the point of injury. Providing the host defences are adequate, no corrective action need be taken. Wound dressing management is aimed at providing an environment for repair.

Colonisation

Bacteria are present and multiplying in the wound but normal host defences are controlling bacterial numbers and there are no negative effects on wound healing.

Critical colonisation

Bacterial numbers have reached a level or toxicity where wound healing is interrupted or delayed. Measures need to be taken to reduce pathogen levels if normal healing is to recommence. Topical antimicrobial dressings, such as silver- or iodine-based products, are indicated in this instance.

Local infection

Pathogen numbers or toxicity is causing deterioration of the local wound environment. Extension of the wound may occur into previously healthy tissue. Topical antimicrobial dressings, or topical antibiotics, may control bacterial growth and improve the wound healing environment. Patients with a poor host defence mechanism may require systemic therapy.

Systemic infection

The wound is deteriorating with spreading cellulitis and systemic signs of infection, such as pyrexia. The patient requires appropriate systemic antimicrobial therapy. Wound management may be geared to the management of the negative effects of infection, such as high exudate levels, pain and odour. Prevention of cross-infection to other individuals is of high importance. Dressings must be able to manage strike-through.

Patients may progress along the Infection Continuum at differing rates (*Figure 2.7*). White (2003) describes how the individual's risk of infection is likened to a balance. On one side is the individual's defence mechanism or immunocompetence and, on the other, is the load on the wound. This load is composed of the number and virulence of the pathogens, and the potentiators of infection such as necrotic burden or the presence of foreign bodies. Alternatively, this can be described as an equation:

$$I = \frac{V \times N}{HDM}$$

Where   I equals infection
V equals virulence of the pathogen
N equals the number or dose of the organism
HDM equals the host defence mechanism

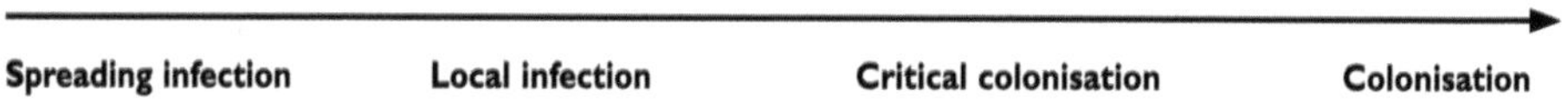

| Spreading infection | Local infection | Critical colonisation | Colonisation |

Figure 2.7: The Wound Infection Continuum (Gray *et al*, 2005)

In either of these instances, it can be seen that the clinician's role is to optimise the body's normal defence mechanisms while reducing the influence that the pathogen has on the individual. This can be achieved by ensuring that bacterial contamination of the wound is minimised with good infection control measures and, where necessary, reducing loading through the use of antimicrobials.

The role of antibiotics

Wound infections have significant, if not life-threatening consequences for patients. Management is essential. As already stated, antibiotics have a key role in the treatment of major wound infections.However, the advent of bacterial resistance has lead to a re-evaluation of their role. Antibiotics need to be considered as 'designer drugs'. Each family of drugs has a specific action on specific cellular functions of certain bacterial groups, and so, no one drug is effective against all organisms. In addition, some pathogens, such as viruses or fungi, remain unaffected by antibiotics due to their cellular make-up. In these cases, specific alternative drug therapies need to be employed.

Successful use of antibiotics is achieved when the appropriate drug is delivered in adequate amounts to achieve elimination of the pathogen. Broad-spectrum antibiotics should be used where the causative organism is unknown and until such time as it can be identified from culture. Once isolated, sensitivity testing can identify the appropriate specific antibiotic to treat the infection. Factors such as poor blood flow due to vascular disease, poor patient concordance in administration of medication, or the presence of necrotic tissue, can reduce the effectiveness of antibiotic regimes. These need to be corrected or compensated for when prescribing treatment.

Topical antibiotics can be a particular problem as their positive action may be neutralised or reduced by the inability to measure and control dosage, the diluting effects of wound exudate, and their reduced ability to permeate debris such as slough and necrotic tissue. Topical antibiotics need to be delivered in a base carrier compound that is able to ensure even distribution over the wound bed. Aqueous preparations can be applied to moist surfaces, but the use of a petroleum-based ointment may prohibit even application. Some preparations may need frequent reapplications to maintain effectiveness, eg. mupirocin. This can prove problematic where reapplication is compromised by the need to maintain wound dressings.

Indiscriminate use of antibiotics leads to bacterial adaptation and the emergence of resistant strains. This complicates treatment not only for the individual concerned, but also for subsequent individuals exposed to the organism. Therefore, their use needs to be targeted at scenarios where other measures would be ineffective. Such scenarios include systemic and spreading infection, and cases where individuals are immunocompromised.

The use of antimicrobials

A number of preparations are available that have a toxic effect on a number of pathogens by simultaneously interfering with a number of cellular functions. Historically, these have been known as antiseptics. Nowadays though, this term tends to be reserved for solutions that are used as disinfectants on intact skin or damaged tissues. These include preparations such as alcohols, hydrogen peroxide and chlorinated solutions (eg. EUSOL). These products have a broad action and can be highly effective in destroying pathogens but may compromise healthy tissues (Morgan, 1997). Their use tends to be questionable in the ongoing management of wounds, and their indications tend to be limited to reduction of pathogen load on intact skin.

Recent advances in antiseptic technology have resulted in the development of products that are relatively harmless to healthy tissue, but which have profound effects on pathogens. Collectively, these products are known as antimicrobials (although antibiotics can also be classified as such). These can be used successfully in topical mode to reduce the loading of a wide variety of pathogens, not only bacteria. Foremost among these are the iodine- and silver-containing preparations.

Iodine

Iodine is a potent antimicrobial agent, however, in its elemental form, it is toxic to mammalian tissues. Subsequent development of povidone-iodine products reduced its toxic effects while maintaining its beneficial effects on pathogenic organisms. It can be delivered as a solution or, more commonly, as a non-adherent dressing (Inadine™ [Johnson and Johnson]) where it rapidly 'dumps' active compounds. Here it can be effective at reducing the effects of heavy local colonisation. It is, however, neutralised by the presence of exudate and is rapidly inactivated in moist wounds. Binding iodine to starch molecules, as in cadexomer iodine (eg. Iodoflex™ [Smith and Nephew] and Iodosorb™ [Smith and Nephew]), extends the duration of antimicrobial effect, as well as providing additional absorbent potential. In both cases it should be noted that sensitivity and systemic absorption could occur. Clinicians must ensure that these products are not used on patients with a known allergy to iodine or pre-existing thyroid dysfunction, and that prolonged therapy is avoided.

Silver

It is argued that the beneficial effects of silver in reducing pathogenic organisms has been recognised throughout history (White, 2003). The new-found interest in silver as an antimicrobial in wound care has led to the emergence of a plethora of products over the past few years. Like iodine, silver acts in many different ways to inhibit pathogenic proliferation. For example, it:

- interferes with the internal transport mechanisms
- binds to DNA, stabilising it and impairing cell division
- damages the cell wall
- damages receptor functionality on cell wall and, thus, membrane transport
- reduces metabolic activity by forming insoluble compounds from otherwise active components) (White and Cooper, 2003).

This makes it a useful treatment option in the management of bacterial load. It can be delivered in a variety of methods and compounds: silver sulfadiazine cream (Flamazine™ [Smith and Nephew]) and tulle (Urgotulle SSD™ [Parema]), nano crystalline silver (Acticoat™ [Smith and Nephew]) and silver compound dressings (Aquacel AG™ [ConvaTec], Contreet™ [Coloplast], Actisorb 220™ [Johnson and Johnson]).

When assessing the effectiveness of each of these products, the clinician needs to evaluate the product's method of silver delivery, ability to deliver silver, quantity and sustainability of silver delivery, suitability for clinical and technical use and, most importantly, clinical outcome.

Conclusion

In most cases, the clinician can effectively modulate the wound environment to achieve positive endpoints for patients, provided that they have a clear understanding of what they want to achieve, have set realistic and measurable outcome objectives, and are fully conversant with the products and technologies that they wish to employ. This last element is one where all clinicians have a duty to maintain and develop their own level of knowledge and competence. This can be achieved by the assimilation of research findings and publications, manufacturers' technical data and guidance, fellow clinicians' findings and recommendations, and personal experience.

References

Ayello EA, Baranoski S, Kerstein MD, Cuddigan J (2004) Wound debridement. In: *Wound Care Essentials: Practice principles.* Springhouse, Lippincott Williams & Wilkins

Baharestani M (eds) (1999) *The Clinical Relevance of Debridement.* Springer, Berlin

Beldon P (2004) Skin grafts. In: White R, ed. *Trends in Wound Care, volume III.* Quay Books, MA Healthcare Ltd, London

Cuzzell JZ (1988) The new red, yellow, black color code. *Am J Nurs* **88**(10) 1342–46

Dunford C (1999) Hypergranulation tissue. *J Wound Care* **8**(10): 506–7

Gray D, White R, Cooper P, Kingsley A (2005) Understanding applied wound management. *Wounds UK* **1**(1): 62–8

Hampton S (1997) Wound assessment. *Prof Nurse* **12**(12): 57

Harris A, Rolstad BS (1994) Hypergranulation tissue; a non-traumatic method of management. *Ostomy/Wound Management* **40**: 20–30

Kingsley A (2005) Practical use of modern honey dressings in chronic wounds. In: White R, Cooper R, Molan P, eds. *Honey: A modern wound management product.* Wounds UK, Aberdeen

Krasner D (1995) Wound care: how to use the red-yellow-black system. *Am J Nurs* **95**(5) 44–7

Leaper D (2002) Sharp technique for wound debridement. Available online at: http://www.worldwidewounds.com/2002/december/Leaper/Sharp-Debridement.html

Molan P (2005) Mode of action. In: White R, Cooper R, Molan P, eds. *Honey: A modern wound management product.* Wounds UK, Aberdeen

Morgan D (1997) *Formulary of Wound Management Products.* 7th edn. Euromed Communications Ltd, Surrey

O'Brien M (2003) Exploring methods of wound debridement. In: White R, ed. *Trends in Wound Care, volume II.* Quay Books, MA Healthcare Ltd, London

Ovington L (2002) Hanging wet-to-dry dressings out to dry. *Adv Skin Woundcare* **15**(2): 79–84

Palmier S, Trial C (2004) Use of high pressure waterjets in wound debridement. In: Teot L, Banwell PE, Ziegler U, eds. _Surgery in Wounds_. Springer-Verlag, Berlin

Ramundo J, Wells J (2000) Wound debridement. In: Bryant, ed. _Acute and Chronic Wounds: Nursing Management_. Mosby, St Louis

Stephen-Haynes J (2005) Implications of honey dressings within primary care. In: White R, Cooper R, Molan P, eds. _Honey: A modern wound management product_. Wounds UK, Aberdeen

Thomas AM, Harding KG, Moore K (1999) The structure and composition of chronic wound eschar. _J Wound Care_ **8**: 258–87

Thomas S, Andrews AM, Hay NP, Bourgoise S (1999) The antimicrobial activity of maggot secretions: results of a preliminary study. _J Tissue Viability_ **9**(4): 127–32

Thomas S (2001) Sterile maggots and the preparation of the wound bed. In: Cherry GW, Harding KG, Ryan TJ, eds. Wound Bed Preparation International Congress and symposium series 250. The Royal Society of Medicine Press, London

Tong A (1999) The identification and treatment of slough. _J Wound Care_ **8**(7): 338–9

Vowden P (2004) Autolytic debridement. In Teot L, Banwell PE, Ziegler U, eds. _Surgery in Wounds_. Springer-Verlag, Berlin

Vowden KR, Vowden P (1999) Wound debridement, Part 1: non-sharp techniques. _J Wound Care_ **8**(5): 237–40

Vowden KR, Vowden P (2002) Wound bed preparation. Available online at: http://www.worldwidewounds.com/2002/april/Vowden/Wound-Bed-Preparation.html

White RJ (2003) The wound infection continuum. In: White R, ed. _Trends in Wound Care, volume II_. Quay Books, MA Healthcare Ltd, London

White R (2003) An historical overview of the use of silver in wound management. In: White R, ed. _The Silver Book_. Quay Books, MA Healthcare Ltd, London

White R, Cooper R (2003) The use of topical antimicrobials in wound bioburden control. In: White R, ed. _The Silver Book_. Quay Books, MA Healthcare Ltd, London

Young T (1995) Common problems in overgranulation. _Practice Nurse_ **6**(11): 14–16

Young T (1997) Use of a hydrocolloid in overgranulation. _J Wound Care_ **6**(5): 216

WOUND PROGRESSION MODEL

CAUSE	PROGRESSION TO HEALING	SYMPTOM MANAGEMENT
BEFORE DECIDING ON ANY TREATMENT PLAN, AN UNDERSTANDING OF THE WOUND'S CAUSE IS REQUIRED	THE PRESENCE OF NECROTIC, SLOUGHY TISSUE, OR INFECTION, CAN DELAY THE PROGRESSION TO HEALING	THE MANAGEMENT OF SYMPTOMS ASSOCIATED WITH WOUNDS SUCH AS THOSE LISTED BELOW CAN BE FACILITATED BY THE CORRECT SELECTION OF PRODUCTS

CAUSE

- LEG ULCER
- DIABETIC FOOT ULCER
- PRESSURE ULCER
- BURN
- SURGICAL WOUND
- TRAUMATIC WOUND

PROGRESSION TO HEALING

REMOVE NECROSIS	REMOVE SLOUGH	MANAGE INFECTION

PROMOTE GRANULATION

DELAYED HEALING, KICK-START HEALING

PROMOTE EPITHELIALISATION

SYMPTOM MANAGEMENT

- ODOUR
- PAIN
- BLEEDING
- EXUDATE
  >HIGH   >MEDIUM   >LOW

Chapter 3

Symptom management

Sue Bale

Although achieving complete wound closure or healing is the ultimate aim of many wound interventions, other factors are also considered important, in particular, the control of wound symptoms. Research that examines the patient experience indicates that odour, exudate, pain and bleeding are the key symptoms that patients find difficult to tolerate (Edwards, 2003; Vowden and Vowden, 2004). As well as the physical discomfort related to these symptoms, patients can also be affected at a personal level. The frequency and extent to which clinicians caring for patients with wounds consider the impact of those wounds on the patient as an individual has been questioned (Baharestani, 2004). Baharestani argues that equal importance should be assigned to the meaning and significance of a wound for individual patients, as is currently assigned to the routine assessment of wound size and wound bed condition. Chronic wounds have been reported to have dramatic effects on patients' lives, and can also result in many challenges as patients struggle to cope with these chronic wounds (Neil and Munjas, 2000). In addition, Baharestani (2004) describes research that has highlighted how some healthcare professionals can have a negative image of patients with chronic wounds, viewing them as unattractive, imperfect, vulnerable, a nuisance and, occasionally, even repulsive. Although these issues need addressing through education and training, many clinicians are striving to attain the best quality of care possible for patients that experience wound healing problems. Indeed, the delivery of wound care that is of a high standard, evidence-based and patient-focused is high on the agenda of many of those caring for patients with wounds.

Careful consideration and appropriate management of wound symptoms that affect the individual are key to patient-centred wound care. This chapter explores these symptoms, what they are, why they occur, and how they can be managed to guide the wound care practitioner towards better practice by employing evidence-based practice.

Odour

Many aetiologies of wounds are associated with odour, particularly chronic pressure ulcers, leg ulcers, ischaemic wounds and fungating malignant ulcers (Benbow, 1999; Holloway *et al*, 2002). The physiological pathway that leads to odour is not yet fully understood, but it is postulated to involve infection, anaerobic bacterial colonisation, tissue degradation and necrosis, either in isolation or in combination (Benbow, 1999; Collier, 2001; Holloway *et al*, 2002; Thomas *et al*, 1998).

Malodorous wounds have been defined as those identified by patients or practitioners as having an offensive smell (Neal, 1991). Olfactory receptors in the nose detect and recognise smells, registering them across a continuum from pleasant to unpleasant. There is a universal aversion connected to malodours associated with decomposition that evokes 'primordial reactions' as a protective mechanism against ingesting, or being in contact with, dangerous bacteria (Van Toller, 1993). Owing to the importance attached to odour, malodorous wounds can have a profound effect on a patient's quality of life (Griep *et al*, 1997). This is particularly the case for anaerobic bacteria, which emit the compounds putrescine, cadaverine, votaltile sulphur compounds, and short-chain fatty acids (Holloway *et al*, 2002). *Pseudomonas* and *Klebsiella* are two species of aerobic bacteria that produce an acrid malodour and these bacteria can cause, at the extreme, a vomit or gag reflex (Van Toller, 1993). Negative effects associated with living with chronic malodorous wounds include: altered body image, feelings of rejection, shame and embarrassment, social withdrawal, reduced appetite, depression, inhibition of intimacy, and social isolation (Boardman *et al*, 1993; Clark, 1992; Grocott, 2000; Hack, 2003; Neal, 1991; Price, 1996). Malodour can also affect nurses. Wilkes *et al* (2003) explored the difficulties nurses faced in caring for patients with malignant malodorous wounds, reporting that the nurses included in their study strove to provide the best care for patients and their relatives under circumstances that they often found physically and emotionally difficult. This was the case whether the patient was aware or not of the malodour.

Interpretation of malodour, and discrepancies in perceptions of the level and intensity of malodour, has also been demonstrated to be problematic as individuals have different thresholds (Wilkes *et al*, 2003). Some patient groups are prone to being unaware of malodour. Odour perception may decline in elderly people (Larsson and Blackman, 1997), as well as in those with ill health or poor nutritional state (Griep *et al*,

1997). The body can protect an individual from being saturated by weak stimuli (such as odours) by desensitising sensory cells, leading the patient to have a weaker odour perception (Gold and Pugh, 1997). There are a number of ways to manage this difficult clinical problem:

❖ *Systemic antibiotics:* not all odour will indicate the presence of infection, but where infection is deep-seated and caused by pathogenic organisms, the use of systemic antibiotics can be indicated. The type of antibiotic will be driven by the organism and the route will depend on the severity of infection and the health of the individual patient.

❖ *Topical antibiotics:* over the past ten years, topical metronidazole, in the form of an aqueous gel, has become an increasingly popular treatment for malodorous wounds. Topical metronidazole acts by binding to bacterial DNA, thus interfering with its replication, eradicating malodour within seven days (Bale *et al*, 2004; Bower *et al*, 1992; McMullen, 1992).

❖ *Topical antimicrobial agents:* applied directly onto the wound bed these active agents include silver ions and cadexomer iodine that reduces bacteria (*Chapter 2, pp. 33, 42–43*).They are available as primary contact materials or as secondary pads.

❖ *Honey:* more recently, honey has been demonstrated to reduce odour by suppressing microbial growth and eliminating bacteria. Pathogenic bacteria metabolise glucose rather than amino acids and so malodorous compounds fail to form. Honey also produces hydrogen peroxide, stimulates an immune response, and supplies glucose for macrophage activity (Dunford, 2005).

❖ *Charcoal:* activated charcoal dressings contain a layer of charcoal that binds the molecules responsible for odour (Miller, 1998). There are a number of products, some are plain activated charcoal cloth (CliniSorb® [Clinimed]), others combine absorbent wound contact layers (CarboFlex® [ConvaTec], Lyofoam C™ [Medlock Medical]), and others contain antimicrobial agents (Actisorb® Silver 220 [J&J]).

For many patients, having a malodorous wound is a devastating life event. This is compounded when patients are also experiencing terminal illness or distressing chronic wounds, such as pressure and leg ulcers. Selecting the most suitable treatment for malodour is essential for ensuring that patients have the optimal quality of life.

Necrosis and slough

Dead, non-viable tissue consists of dead cells, debris, fibrin and pus (*pp. 22–23*). As a symptom, the presence of sloughy, necrotic, devitalised tissue on the wound bed can cause malodour as it degrades. Due to the adverse effect of malodour on patients, it is important to resolve it quickly (*pp. 47–48*). Necrosis and slough also provides an ideal medium to support bacterial growth (Schultz *et al*, 2004), and could lead to wound infection. To reduce the bioburden of the wound and to control or prevent infection, it is important to remove devitalised tissue as quickly and efficiently as possible (Ayello *et al*, 2004). However, this can be difficult to achieve, as when both slough and necrotic tissue are firmly stuck to the wound bed, they cannot simply be wiped away. There are several ways of achieving wound debridement.

Surgical/sharp debridement

Surgical or sharp debridement using a scalpel, forceps, scissors or laser is by far the quickest and most effective method, as debridement is immediate and a healthy wound bed can result. Here, the devitalised or dead tissue is cut away from the healthy tissue by an experienced and competent practitioner who is knowledgeable about the anatomy of the area being debrided (Ayello *et al*, 2004). Thorough and effective surgical debridement down to healthy, viable tissue is best undertaken by a doctor with surgical skills, or a specially trained nurse, as some bleeding usually results (Ramundo and Wells, 2000). In the UK, Fairbairn *et al* (2002) developed a framework for knowledge and competency-based practice to provide guidelines for nurses wishing to undertake sharp debridement. It is not always feasible or practical to undertake sharp or surgical debridement. For example, if patients are being cared for in the community, an experienced and competent practitioner may not be available, or their physical environment may be unsuitable, and so a conservative approach will be required.

Autolytic debridement

When exposed to a moist environment, devitalised tissue undergoes a natural process of autolysis where phagocytes and proteolytic enzymes soften and liquefy devitalised tissue, which is then digested by macrophages (Ayello _et al_, 2004). Modern wound dressings, including hydrogels and hydrocolloids, will provide a moist wound environment that facilitates autolysis (_Chapter 2, p. 24_).

Enzymatic debridement

This is achieved by applying topical enzymatic agents to the devitalised tissue, where they chemically digest and dissolve this tissue (Ramundo and Wells, 2000).

Larval therapy

Larvae digest devitalised tissue by secreting proteolytic enzymes onto the wound bed, liquefying and breaking down dead tissue. Larvae ingest the liquefied tissue and other debris and bacteria (_Chapter 2, p. 27_).

Honey

As well as providing a moist environment conducive to autolysis, honey has an additional benefit of drawing fluid from the surrounding tissues, thus facilitating protease activity at the interface between healthy and devitalised tissue (White and Molan, 2005).

Infection

Wound malodour is frequently associated with infection, as bacteria multiply and produce pus. Whether or not a wound infection develops depends on the nature of the host's resistance, in combination with the degree of pathogenicity and number of the invading bacteria (Bowler, 2002). Although most wounds are colonised with a mixture of bacteria, when pathogenic bacteria invade the wound bed and surrounding tissues the clinical signs of infection become apparent. With respect to wound bed infection, these signs include red, bleeding, flimsy, friable and painful granulation tissue (Cutting and White, 2004). For deeper tissue infection, erythema, oedema, pain, odour and purulent exudate are also included (Gardner and Frantz, 2004). Surgical wound infection has been defined as one that occurs at the site of surgery within thirty days of surgery or within one year if an implant has been inserted (Stotts, 2000). It can be categorised as superficial, involving only the skin and subcutaneous tissue of the incision, or deep, involving the deep soft tissues (Gardener and Frantz, 2004).

Exudate

Exudate is the fluid that wounds produce. Assessment of its volume, viscosity and appearance indicate the health status of a wound and typically influence the practitioner's choice of dressing and/or other intervention. Control of exudate to ensure that a balance between too much and too little is achieved presents practitioners with real clinical challenges. The key aim of symptom control is to optimise exudate levels, protect the surrounding skin, and maximise patients' quality of life by preventing leakage, controlling odour and reducing pain (Cutting, 2004; Vowden and Vowden, 2004). Modern wound care interventions, including dressings, have been designed to balance the levels of wound exudate (Bishop *et al*, 2003).

Exudate has a high content of protein, with cellular debris, bacteria and leukocytes (Baranoski and Ayello, 2004), which indicate health or the presence of disease. Healthy wound exudate is rich in enzymes and growth factors (Bates-Jensen, 1998), whereas unhealthy exudate is associated with inappropriate or defective cellular and cytokine activity (Hart, 2002; Moore, 1999; Park *et al*, 1998). As with other aspects of wound care, it is important that practitioners managing wounds are able to identify and distinguish between normality and abnormality. Cutting (2004) argues that exudate is too often perceived as a problem in clinical practice, and that it should be accepted as a mostly beneficial element of normal wound healing. When healthy exudate bathes a wound, it provides a moist environment in which healing can proceed. Achieving the optimal level of exudate is a challenge as too much can cause maceration and skin breakdown, whereas too little leads to dehydration and desiccation of the wound bed.

Healthy wound exudate bathes the wound in:

- essential nutrients and electrolytes (Cutting, 2004)
- growth factors that stimulate and regulate the healing cascade (Moore, 1999)
- cells that control haemostatis, promote debridement and produce growth factors (Waldrop and Doughty, 2000). Neutrophils ingest bacteria and other debris and, in the early stages of healing, cleanse the wound (Cutting, 2004). Later, macrophages take over this function, and also have a major role in stimulating and regulating growth factor produce and synthesis (Waldrop and Doughty, 2000)
- inflammatory components — leukocytes, fibrinogen and fibrin (Cutting, 2004).

Research suggests that exudate from chronic ulceration appears to have a damaging effect on normal wound healing due to continued raised levels of tissue destructive enzymes (Drinkwater *et al*, 2002; Trengrove *et al*, 1996; Wysocki *et al*, 1993). Unhealthy wound exudate bathes the wound in any of, or a combination of:

- inappropriate types or levels of growth factors (Hart, 2002; Wallace and Stacey, 1998)
- high levels of proteases, lactate, low pH and PO2 (Moore, 1999)
- pathogenic bacteria (Bates-Jensen, 1998; Vowden and Vowden, 2002)
- inappropriate lymphocyte and macrophage populations and inappropriate endothelial cell adhesion molecules (Moore, 1999).

Whether healthy or unhealthy, excessive levels of wound exudate can saturate and damage the wound bed and surrounding skin, causing the patient pain and discomfort, as well as considerable inconvenience as moisture seeps through dressings and bandages (Bale, 2000). Where excessive levels of wound exudate are present, it is important to understand whether this is related to a problem that can be resolved, for example, infection or oedema. Where high volumes are associated with a large surface area of wound or deep, extensive tissue loss in otherwise healthy wounds, a number of measures can be taken to contain or control this wound symptom:

* ❖ **Use of absorbent dressing materials:** several dressing materials, such as alginates (Hydrofiber®), foams and combination dressings can be used to control high levels of exudate production (*Chapter 2*). These are highly absorbent products that have been designed to wick or absorb exudate away from the wound bed and surrounding skin, hold moisture in and reduce frequency of dressing changes. To enhance exudate control, some dressings absorb and retain exudate while transmitting moisture through the outer top layer, thus increasing their moisture handling capacity (Bishop *et al*, 2003). In addition, dressings need to be able to provide these properties under a range of different physical conditions, including under compression therapy and in conjunction with pressure-relieving surfaces. Dressing performance has been evaluated from the patient and user perspective by Grocott (1998, 2000) specifically to inform the development of dressings.
* ❖ **Use of topical negative pressure (TNP):** this therapy is designed to control heavily exuding wounds by applying subatmospheric pressure to the wound bed using a sealed system (Broussard *et al*, 2000). Excess exudate is drawn away from the wound bed by a pump and collected in a drainage container. In addition to managing exudate, it has been suggested that topical negative pressure therapy also accelerates wound healing by stimulating angiogenesis, promoting healthy granulation tissue, decreasing bacterial load, removing toxic chemicals and matrix metaloproteinases, and increasing nutrient and oxygen levels (Baranoski and Ayello, 2004; Broussard *et al*, 2000; Vowden and Vowden, 2004).
* ❖ **Increasing frequency of change when appropriate choice of dressing has been made:** there are occasions when despite choosing a highly absorbent dressing, the level of exudate production is so high that leakage occurs before a daily dressing change.

Too little wound exudate can also be problematic as the wound bed dries out, leaving a scab or layer of desiccated exudate. Research has demonstrated that healing is delayed in a dry wound environment in both an animal model (Winter, 1962) and in human skin (Hinman and Maibach, 1963; Eaglestein, 1985). Providing a moist wound environment in experimental conditions doubled the rate of epithelialisation, as epithelial cells migrated more quickly and were unimpeded. Autolytic debridement of dead cells and debris is also enhanced by a moist wound environment (Ramundo and Wells, 2000). Apart from adversely affecting epithelial migration, dry wounds can inhibit the beneficial properties of wound exudate demonstrated to promote healing in acute wounds (Parnham, 2002). Parnham (2002) reviews experimental research where increased numbers of macrophages, fibroblasts, myofibroblasts, and increased granulation tissue and wound contraction were reported in a moist wound environment compared to a dry one.

Where a wound bed has dried out, this can be converted to a moist environment by:

- application of a water-donating dressing, such as a hydrogel (*Chapter 2, p. 25; p. 29*)
- application of an adhesive dressing that prevents the loss of moisture, such as a hydrocolloid or semi-permeable film (*Chapter 2, p. 25; p. 29*).

Pain

Pain can be defined as a feeling of distress, suffering or agony caused by stimulation of specialised nerve endings (Seers, 2000). Experiencing pain is unique to the individual, although it is influenced by age, gender, emotional, social and cultural factors (Casey, 1998; Glynn, 2002). Pain has an important protective role to play in wound care as injured tissues stimulate pain, alerting the individual to tissue damage and inducing rest to allow regeneration (Wulf and Baron, 2003). Pain signals are relayed through the neural network by nociceptors (pain-sensing nerves) to the brain, via complex mechanisms, where pain is interpreted (Glynn, 2002; King, 2003). The assessment and management of wound pain is an essential element of symptom control and one that has in the past been overlooked (King, 2003). However, our knowledge and understanding in this area has increased in recent years (Clay and Chen, 2005; Edwards, 2003; Hopkins and Dealey, 2005; Latarjet, 2002; Moffatt *et al*, 2003).

Assessment of pain

It is important to assess a patient's level of pain prior to selecting a treatment option. This can be achieved in a number of ways. Hofman (2002) recommends using the following list of questions to best understand the nature of, as well as the level of, pain experienced:

❖ ***Palliative/provocative:*** What makes the pain better? What makes the pain worse?
❖ ***Quality:*** What is the pain like? Throbbing, stabbing, sharp, dull?
❖ ***Region and radiation:*** Where is the pain? Where does it spread?
❖ ***Severity:*** Scale of severity (visual analogue scale or verbal rating scale)?
❖ ***Temporal aspects:*** Continuous, intermittent, occasional, time of day (for example, night pain) (Dallam *et al*, 2004).

In wound care, pain is usually described as acute or chronic.

Acute wound pain

With acute wound pain there is typically a relationship between the stimulus and the pain response, as might occur with procedural pain, such as during dressing changes or sharp debridement (Glynn, 2002; King, 2003). In many ways, this 'cause and effect' relationship facilitates pain management, as effective treatment of the cause should result in pain relief.

Chronic wound pain

Chronic wound pain is typically persistent and continuous, and linked to procedures or other events (Dallam *et al*, 2004). Although increasingly recognised as a wound symptom, it is often mismanaged or under-managed (Hofman, 2002). In addition, the patient's experience of tolerating chronic pain highlights the need for such patients to be believed by health professionals, as many patients report perceptions that they are not usually believed (Clark and Iphofen, 2005).

Pain relief can be achieved by:

* *Use of appropriate dressings:* dressing change is one of the most common causes of procedural pain in wound management (King, 2003). Dressings that have dried out and adherence of dressings to the wound bed was cited as the most important factor in causing wound pain at dressing change (Moffatt *et al*, 2003). Dressings that provide a moist wound environment ease removal of dressings and, in so doing, reduce pain at dressing change (Clay and Chen, 2005; Moffatt *et al*, 2003). Appropriate selection of dressings is key to controlling pain as a wound symptom.
* *Use of analgesia:* where pain persists despite the use of appropriate wound dressings, a broad range of analgesics can be effectively used to alleviate pain. The most effective for this indication include non-steroidal anti-inflammatory drugs (NSAIDs), conventional analgesics (ranging from paracetamol to opioids), and unconventional analgesics, such as antidepressants (Glynn, 2002).

NSAIDs are recommended as a first line of treatment, administered on a regular, rather than an, 'as needed' basis (Dallam *et al*, 2004). Caution is required in older people where renal failure is a significant risk. Gastric bleeding is also associated with prolonged use. Opioids are available as oral, oral-transmucosal, rectal, transdermal, subcutaneous and intravenous medication, and come in strengths that vary from mild to very strong (Dallam *et al*, 2004; Latarjet, 2002). Constipation, sedation, nausea, vomiting and itching are among the most common side-effects. Tricyclic antidepressants have been demonstrated to be effective at relieving chronic pain, while also providing a sedative effect that is useful at night (Glynn, 2002).

Bleeding

Apart from infection, the other major cause of bleeding is malignancy, where lesions ulcerate through tissues and infiltrate through the epithelium (Mortimer, 1998). Carcinomas and sarcomas are most likely to result in ulceration and fungation in the latter stages of the disease (Bale and Harding, 2000; Goldberg and McGinn-Byer, 2000). The growth of tumours is a complex process that controls blood flow and tissue oxygenation (Grocott, 2000), and this process can be slow or rapid depending on the nature of the malignancy. Malignant lesions include fungating carcinoma of the breast, fungating lesions of malignant melanoma, and a variety of other extending or fungating wounds. Mortimer (1998) has defined the term 'fungating' as describing a malignancy that has ulcerated and infiltrated through the epithelium. Fungating wounds can result either in a protruding growth or an ulcerating cavity (Carville, 1995). Lesions infiltrate the epithelium and supporting lymph and blood vessels and, as the tumour extends, capillaries rupture leading to tissue hypoxia, breakdown and necrosis. Bleeding may also be present due to either fragile capillary walls or infiltration of the tumour mass into surrounding blood vessels (Regnard and Tempest, 1998).

Improvement in the quality of life of patient and family can be achieved by alleviating the distressing symptom of bleeding (Dunlop, 1998). It is essential to maintain the patient's dignity and self-esteem by supporting both carers and patient in care of the lesion by adopting a positive outlook to management. Bleeding can be controlled by the use of:

* **Haemostatic dressings:** alginates (*Chapter 2*) are particularly useful for arresting the bleeding from fragile vessels as malignant tissue infiltrates and fungates through normal tissues. Often these lesions are in an area that is extremely difficult to dress in terms of keeping the dressing in place, eg. on the chest wall, in the groin, and on the lower limb.
* **Dressings that do not adhere to the wound bed so ensuring that removal does not cause further bleeding:** selecting dressings that do not traumatise the wound bed and can be easily and safely removed is key to the management of bleeding. A broad range of products are available, including silicone-impregnated hydrogels, alginates, and non-adherent products (*Chapter 2*).

Conclusion

This chapter has explored the management of wound symptoms, including odour, exudate, pain and bleeding, explaining what they are, why they occur and providing the evidence upon which to base practice. These symptoms are highlighted by patients as causing them the most problem (Edwards, 2003; Vowden and Vowden, 2004). Alongside effectively managing the physical wound symptoms, it is important that clinicians also effectively manage and seek to control the impact of wound symptoms on the patient as an individual person. The next chapter builds on the theory described in _Chapters 1–3_ and presents a series of flow diagrams that show how the Wound Progression Model can be used in practice.

References

Ayello AE, Baranoski S, Kerstein MD, Cuddigan J (2004) Wound debridement. In: Baranoski S, Ayello AE, eds. _Wound Care Essentials: Practice principles._ Lippincott Williams and Wilkins, Springhouse

Bale S, Harding K (2000) The challenges of specific aetiologies. In: Bale S, Harding KG, Leaper D, eds. _An Introduction to Wounds._ Emap, London

Bale S, Leaper D (2000) Acute wounds. In: Bale S, Harding KG, Leaper D, eds. _An Introduction to Wounds._ Emap, London

Bale S, Tebble N, Price P (2004) A topical metronidazole gel used to treat malodorous wounds. _Br J Nurs_ **13**(11): S4–S11

Baranoski S, Ayello AE (2004) _Wound Care Essentials: Practice principles._ Lippincott Williams and Wilkins, Springhouse

Bates-Jensen BM (1998) Management of exudate and infection. In: Sussman C, Bates-Jensen BM, eds. _Wound Care: A Collborative Practice Manual for Physical Therapists and Nurses._ Aspen Publishers Inc, Maryland

Benbow M (1999) Malodorous wounds: how to improve quality of life. _Nurse Prescriber_ **2**: 43–6

Bishop SM, Walker M, Rogers AA, Chen WYJ (2003) Importance of moisture balance at the wound-dressing interface. _J Wound Care_ **12**(4): 125–8

Boardman M, Meelor K, Neville B (1993) Treating a patient with a heavily exudating malodorous fungating ulcer. _J Wound Care_ **8**(5): 216–8

Bower M, Stein R, Evans TR (1992) A double blind study of the efficacy of metronidazole gel. _Eur J Cancer_ **28A**: 888–9

Bowler P (2002) The role of bacteria in wound healing: research or myth? In: _The Oxford European Wound Healing Course Handbook._ Positif Press, Oxford

Broussard CL, Mendez-Eastamn S, Frantz R (2000) Adjuvant wound therapies. In: Bryant RA, ed. _Acute and Chronic Wounds: Nursing Management._ Mosby Inc, St Louis

Carville K (1995) Caring for cancerous wounds in the community. _J Wound Care_ **4**(2): 46–8

Casey G (1998) The management of pain in wound care. *Nurs Standard* **13**(12): 49–54

Clark L (1992) Caring for fungating tumours. *Nurs Times* **88**(12): 66–70

Clark KA, Iphofen R (2005) Believing the patients with chronic pain: a review of the literature. *Br J Nurs* **14**(9): 490–3

Clay CS, Chen WWJ (2005) Wound pain: the need for a more understanding approach. *J Wound Care* **14**(4): 181–4

Collier M (2001) Malodorous and infected wounds: A patient-centred approach. *The Leg Ulcer Forum J* **14**: 12–14

Cutting KF (2004) Wound exudate: composition and functions. In: White RJ, ed. *Trends in Wound Care, volume III*. Quay Books, MA Healthcare Limited, London

Cutting KF, White RJ (2004) Criteria for wound infection by indication. In: White RJ, ed. *Trends in Wound Care, volume III*. Quay Books, MA Healthcare Limited, London

Dallam LE, Barkauskas C, Ayello EA, Baranoski S et al (2004) Pain management and wounds. In: Baranoski S, Ayello AE, eds. *Wound Care Essentials: Practice principles*. Lippincott Williams and Wilkins, Springhouse

Drinkwater SL, Smith A, Sawyer BM, Barnard KG (2002) Effect of venous ulcer exudates on angiogenesis in vitro. *Br J Surg* **89**(6): 709–13

Dunford C (2005) The use of honey in wound management. In: White R, Cooper R, Molan P, eds. *Honey: A modern wound management product* Wounds UK Ltd, Aberdeen

Dunlop R (1998) *Cancer: Palliative Care*. Springer, London

Edwards LM (2003) Why patients do not comply with compression bandages. *Br J Nurs* **12**(11): S5–S16

Fairbairn K, Grier J, Hunter C, Preece J (2002) A sharp debridement procedure devised by specialist nurses. *J Wound Care* **11**(10): 371–5

Gardener SE, Frantz RA (2004) Wound bioburden. In: Baranoski S, Ayello AE, eds. *Wound Care Essentials: Practice principles*. Lippincott Williams and Wilkins, Springhouse

Glynn C (2002) The Control of Pain Associated with Wounds. In: *The Oxford European Wound Healing Course Handbook*. Positif Press, Oxford

Gold GH, Pugh EN (1997) The nose leads the eye. *Nature* **385**: 677–9

Goldberg MT, McGinn-Byer P (2000) Oncology-related skin damage. In: Bryant RA, ed. *Acute and Chronic Wounds: Nursing Management*. Mosby Inc, St Louis

Griep M, Mets RF, Vogalaere P, Collys K, Laska M, Massart DL (1997) Odour perception in relation to age, general health, nutritional status and dental status. *Tijdschr Gerontol Geriatric* **28**(1): 1–7

Grocott P (1998) Exudate management of fungating wounds. *J Wound Care* **7**(9): 445–8

Grocott P (2000) The palliative management of fungating malignant wounds. *J Wound Care* **9**(1): 4–9

Hack A (2003) Malorodous wounds — taking the patient's perspectives into account. *J Wound Care* **12**(8): 319–21

Hart J (2002) Inflammation 2: its role in the healing of chronic wounds. *J Wound Care* **11**: 245–9

Hinman CD, Maibach HI (1963) Effect of air exposure and occlusion on experimental human skin wounds. *Nature* **200**: 377

Hofman D (2002) Practical pain management associated with wounds. In: *The Oxford European Wound Healing Course Handbook*. Positif Press, Oxford

Holloway S, Bale S, Harding KG, Robinson B, Ballard K (2002) Evaluating the effectiveness of a dressing for use in malodorous, exuding wounds. *Ostomy/Wound Management* **48**(5): 22–8

Hopkins A, Dealey C (2005) *The lived experience of pressure ulcers*. 8th European Pressure Ulcer Advisory Panel open meeting, 5–7 May. Aberdeen, Scotland

King B (2003) A review of research investigating pain and wound care. *J Wound Care* **12**(6): 219–23

Krasner D (2000) Managing wound pain. In: Bryant RA, ed. *Acute and Chronic Wounds: Nursing Management*. Mosby Inc, St Louis

Larsson M, Blackman L (1997) Age-related differences in episodic odour recognition the role of access to specific odour names. *Memory* **5**(3): 361–78

Latarjet J (2002) The management of pain associated with dressing changes in patients with burns. *EWMA J* **2**(2): 59

McMullen D (1992) Topical metronidazole: Part II. *Ostomy/Wound Management* **38**(3): 42–8

Moffatt CJ, Franks PJ, Hollinworth H (2003) Understanding wound pain and trauma: an international perspective. In: *Pain at Wound Dressing Changes*. MEP Ltd, London

Moore K (1999) Cell biology of chronic wounds: the role of inflammation. *J Wound Care* **8**(7): 345–8

Mortimer PS (1998) Management of skin problems: medical aspects. In: Doyle D, Hanks GWC, MacDonald N, eds. *Oxford Textbook of Palliative Medicine*. 2nd edn. Oxford University Press, Oxford

Neal K (1991) Treating fungating lesions. *Nurs Times* **87**(23): 85–6

Park HY, Shon K, Phillips T (1998) The effect of heat on the inhibitory effects of chronic wound fluid on fibroblasts in vitro. *Wounds* **10**: 189–92

Parnham A (2002) Moist wound healing: does the theory apply to chronic wounds? *J Wound Care* **11**(4): 143–6

Price E (1996) The stigma of smell. *J Wound Care Nursing, Nurs Times* **92**(20): 71–2

Ramundo J, Wells J (2000) Wound debridement. In: Bryant RA, ed. *Acute and Chronic Wounds: Nursing Management.* Mosby, St Louis

Regnard CF, Tempest S (1998) *A Guide to Symptom Relief in Advanced Cancer.* 4th edn. Hochland and Hochland, Cheshire

Schultz GS, Barillo DJ, Moringo DW, Chin GA (2004) Wound bed preparation and a brief history of TIME. *Int Wound J* **1**(1): 19–32

Seers K (2000) Pain. In: Alexander MF, Fawcett JN, Runciman PJ, eds. *Nursing Practice: Hospital and Home. The Adult.* 2nd edn. Churchill Livingstone, Edinburgh

Stotts NA (2000) Wound infection: diagnosis and management. In: Bryant RA, ed. *Acute and Chronic Wounds: Nursing Management.* Mosby Inc, St Louis

Thomas S, Fisher B, Fram PJ, Waring MJ (1998) Odour-absorbing dressings. *J Wound Care* **7**(5): 246–50

Trengrove N, Langton SR, Stacey MC (1996) Biochemical analysis of wound fluid from non-healing and healing chronic leg ulcers. *Wound Rep Regen* **4**: 234–9

Van Toller S (1993) Psychological consequences arising from the malodours produced by skin ulcers. In: Harding KG, Cherry G, Dealey C, Turner TD, eds. *Proceedings of the 2nd European Conference on Advances in Wound Management.* Macmillan Magazines Ltd, London

Vowden K, Vowden P (2002) Wound bed preparation. Available online at: http://www.worldwidewounds.com (accessed 27.05.05)

Vowden K, Vowden P (2004) The role of exudate in the healing process: understanding exudate management. In: White RJ, ed. *Trends in Wound Care, volume III.* Quay Books, MA Healthcare Limited, London

Waldrop J, Doughty D (2000) Wound-healing physiology. In: Bryant RA, ed. *Acute and Chronic Wounds: Nursing Management.* Mosby Inc, St Louis

Wallace HJ, Stacey MC (1998) Levels of tumour necrosis factor-alpha (TNF-alpha) and soluble TNF receptors in chronic venous leg ulcers — correlations to healing status. *J Investigative Dermatol* **110**(3): 292–6

White R, Molan P (2005) A summary of published clinical research on honey in wound management. In: White RJ, Cooper R, Molan P. eds. *Honey: A modern wound management product.* Wounds UK Ltd, Aberdeen

Wilkes LM, Boxer E, White K (2003) The hidden side of nursing: why caring for patients with malignant malodorous wounds is so difficult. *J Wound Care* **12**(2): 76–80

Winter GD (1962) Formation of the scab and the rate of epithelialization of superficial wounds in the skin of young domestic pigs. *Nature* **193**: 293–4

Wulf H, Baron R (2003) The theory of pain. In: *Pain at Wound Dressing Changes*. MEP Ltd, London

Wysocki AB, Staiano-Coico L, Grinnell F (1993) Wound fluid from chronic leg ulcers contains elevated levels of metallproteinases MMP-2 and MMP-9. *J Investigative Dermatol* **101**: 64–8

WOUND PROGRESSION MODEL

CAUSE

BEFORE DECIDING ON ANY TREATMENT PLAN, AN UNDERSTANDING OF THE WOUND'S CAUSE IS REQUIRED

LEG ULCER

DIABETIC FOOT ULCER

PRESSURE ULCER

BURN

SURGICAL WOUND

TRAUMATIC WOUND

PROGRESSION TO HEALING

THE PRESENCE OF NECROTIC, SLOUGHY TISSUE, OR INFECTION, CAN DELAY THE PROGRESSION TO HEALING

| REMOVE NECROSIS | REMOVE SLOUGH | MANAGE INFECTION |

PROMOTE GRANULATION

DELAYED HEALING, KICK-START HEALING

PROMOTE EPITHELIALISATION

SYMPTOM MANAGEMENT

THE MANAGEMENT OF SYMPTOMS ASSOCIATED WITH WOUNDS SUCH AS THOSE LISTED BELOW CAN BE FACILITATED BY THE CORRECT SELECTION OF PRODUCTS

ODOUR

PAIN

BLEEDING

EXUDATE
>HIGH   >MEDIUM   >LOW

CHAPTER 4

FLOW DIAGRAMS

Sue Bale

Previous chapters have provided an account of wound care with respect to the Wound Progression Model. This model provides a structured framework in which to plan and deliver wound care, identifying the expected logical progression of different wounds.

Pressure ulcers, traumatic and surgical wounds, leg ulcers and diabetic foot ulcers are included for necrotic, sloughy, infected, granulating and epithelialising tissue types. Burns are not included, as these are a specialist aetiology covered by specialist publications on this topic.

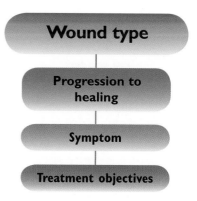

Guide to flow diagrams

Each different wound aetiology and tissue condition clearly defines the possible pathways that patients might take. The case scenarios describe the patient and their settings, presenting the clinical challenges faced by nurses as they assess and decide on treatment options. This is followed by a route through the flow diagram for managing each case, demonstrating how you can use these diagrams for your patients with their own clinical challenges in your clinical setting. The rationale is given for decision choices to help the reader understand how and why these decisions were made.

This chapter consolidates the learning from previous chapters, bringing to life the theory and illustrating how it can be used to deliver evidence-based practice.

Pressure ulcer — necrotic

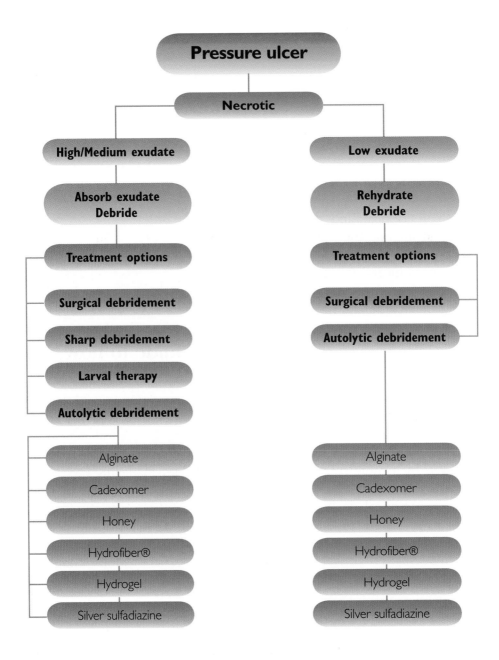

Case scenario

Betty Woods is an eighty-two-year-old retired teacher who has been living in a care home for four years. Prior to this she was fiercely independent and had an active social life. All this gradually came to an end when she developed Alzheimer's disease, deteriorated physically and mentally, and was admitted to a care home. During the past six months Betty's condition has deteriorated even further and she has been confined to bed and had numerous hospital admissions. She has lost weight, been immobile in bed, incontinent of urine and faeces and started to develop contractures. A large, grade 4 sacral pressure ulcer has developed, that comprises mostly necrotic tissue (_Figure 4.1_). A nursing assessment highlighted a Waterlow score of 25. It also detected that she was nutritionally depleted and had an additional risk of skin breakdown due to incontinence. She also requires physiotherapy for her joints. Although her pain level was difficult to assess, the nurses thought that she had procedural pain at dressing changes and she was, at this time, the most sick and dependent patient in the care home. Betty's care plan reflected her needs and provided: a low air loss bed with regular repositioning; help with feeding and additional nutritional support; skin care; pain relief prior to dressings; and physiotherapy with additional nursing care to help mobilise her joints. Wound assessment identified a grade 4 pressure ulcer, mostly filled with dry, necrotic tissue. There was little odour and no clinical signs of infection, but Betty was experiencing procedural pain as the alginate packing used was adherent to the wound bed and difficult to remove. The first priority of local wound care was to debride the wound of necrotic tissue.

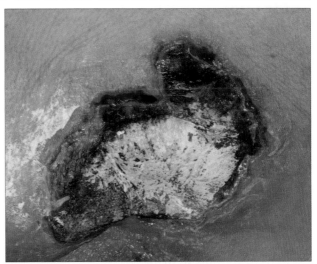

Figure 4.1: Grade 4 sacral pressure ulcer

The following pathway through the flow diagram was selected.

Necrotic

Necrosis comprises dead, non-viable tissue made up of dead cells, debris, fibrin and pus, providing an ideal medium to support bacterial growth (Schultz *et al*, 2004). It is important to remove devitalised tissue as quickly and efficiently as possible to reduce the bioburden of the wound and to control or prevent infection (Ayello *et al*, 2004). This can be difficult as when necrotic tissue is firmly stuck to the wound bed it cannot simply be wiped away.

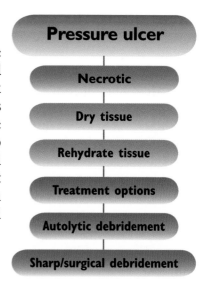

Dry tissue

Too little wound exudate can also be problematic as the wound bed dries out, leaving a scab or layer of desiccated exudate. Research has demonstrated that healing is delayed in a dry wound environment in both an animal model (Winter, 1962) and in human skin (Eaglestein, 1985; Hinman and Maibach, 1963). With necrotic tissue, the devitalised tissue has died and formed a hard, leathery eschar. A dry wound environment can inhibit the beneficial properties of wound exudate, which promotes healing by increasing numbers of macrophages, fibroblasts, and myofibroblasts. Increased granulation tissue and wound contraction have been reported in a moist wound environment compared to a dry one (Parnham, 2002).

Rehydrate and debride

When exposed to a moist environment, devitalised tissue undergoes a natural process of autolysis where phagocytes and proteolytic enzymes soften and liquefy devitalised tissue, which is then digested by macrophages (Ayello *et al*, 2004).

Treatment options ● Autolytic debridement

Modern wound dressings, including hydrogels and hydrocolloids, provide a moist wound environment that facilitates autolysis. Where a wound bed has dried out, this can be converted to a moist environment by:

- application of a water-donating dressing, such as a hydrogel
- application of an adhesive dressing that prevents the loss of moisture, such as a hydrocolloid or semi-permeable film.

In managing Betty, the decision was made to apply a hydrogel and hold it in place with a semi-permeable film dressing, initially changed on a daily basis. The rationale for doing so included:

- ❖ The hydrogel would donate water into the dry necrotic tissue, providing the moist wound environment needed to encourage the natural process of autolytic debridement.
- ❖ Procedural pain would be reduced as the gel is easier to rinse from the wound bed.
- ❖ The use of a semi-permeable film dressing would help to keep moisture from the dressing in contact with the wound bed.
- ❖ The use of a semi-permeable film dressing would help to protect the wound from contamination of urine and faeces during the episodes of incontinence that Betty was experiencing as an ongoing problem.
- ❖ Daily dressing changes were justified to stop the wound bed from drying out. Initially, it was important that some experience was gained from this dressing regime for Betty. It was important that a generous amount of hydrogel was used. This was to be reviewed after a few days, with a view to both decreasing the amount of hydrogel used and the frequency of dressing changes.

Evaluation of Betty's care was undertaken and after nine days much of the necrotic tissue had been rehydrated and was beginning to separate from the wound bed. As this process progressed, increasing odour was noted, although there remained an absence of clinical signs of infection, both locally and systemically. The decision was made to perform sharp debridement of the loose necrotic tissue at the bedside.

Surgical or sharp debridement using a scalpel, forceps, scissors, or laser is by far the quickest and most effective method: debridement is immediate and a healthy wound bed can result. In the UK, Fairbairn _et al_ (2002) developed a framework for knowledge and competency-based practice to provide guidelines for nurses wishing to undertake sharp debridement. Following this procedure, much of the necrotic tissue was removed and over the next twenty-four hours the odour resolved. Dressing changes were carried out on alternate days, and loose pieces of necrotic tissue trimmed away. After a further ten days, most of the necrotic tissue had been removed and Betty's wound care plan was changed accordingly.

Pressure ulcer — sloughy

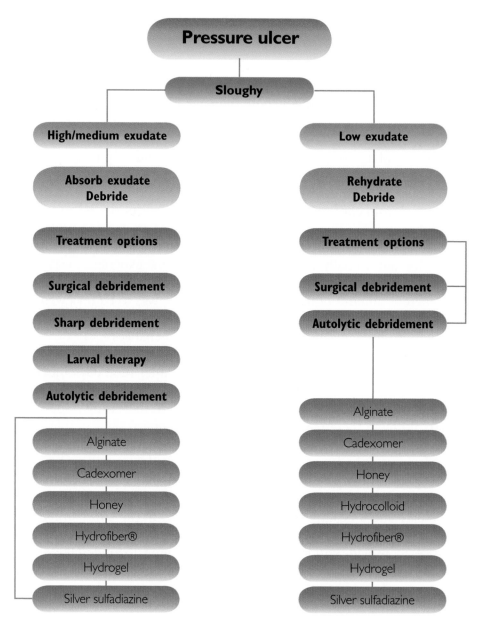

Case scenario

Phillip Watkins is a sixty-seven-year-old retired car mechanic, married for thirty-eight years and living with his wife, who is also retired. Until recently, they have been enjoying an active retirement. Phillip was diagnosed with diabetes fifteen years ago but, despite taking oral hypoglycaemic tablets, he has been struggling to keep control of his blood sugar levels. Following the onset of a severe chest infection, Phillip was admitted to hospital for intravenous antibiotics and was immobile for around a week. During this time, his blood sugar levels were difficult to control, he lost weight, and had his mobility restricted by an infusion pump. A small grade 3 pressure ulcer developed on his left heel, initially as a blister, and then becoming a sloughy lesion. Phillip's general condition improved rapidly, he became mobile and independent, regained his appetite, and went back to his regular oral medication. Phillip's care plan reflected his improved condition, focusing on maintaining control of his diabetes and managing his pressure ulcer. Specifically, he required relief of pressure to his feet with regular repositioning, monitoring of diabetes status and a vascular assessment, and ongoing monitoring of circulation to his foot. It was important to assess whether or not the pressure ulcer was related

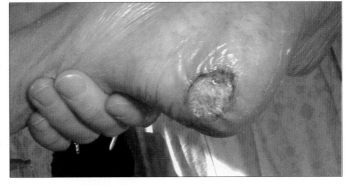

to ischaemia of **Figure 4.2: Grade 3 pressure ulcer to the heal**
the lower limb as a consequence of diabetes. A review by the vascular surgeon and the results of a Duplex scan confirmed that limited ischaemia was present and that it was safe to proceed with wound debridement. Wound assessment had identified a grade 3 pressure ulcer, mostly covered with wet, sloughy tissue (_Figure 4.2_). There was little odour and no clinical signs of infection. The first priority of local wound care was to debride the wound of necrotic tissue.

The following pathway through the flow diagram was selected.

Sloughy

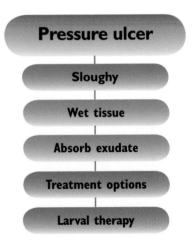

Slough comprises dead, non-viable tissue made up of dead cells, debris, fibrin and pus, providing an ideal medium to support bacterial growth (Schultz *et al*, 2004). To reduce the bioburden of the wound and to control or prevent infection, it is important to remove devitalised tissue as quickly and efficiently as possible (Ayello *et al*, 2004). This can be difficult as when sloughy tissue is firmly stuck to the wound bed it cannot simply be wiped away.

Pressure ulcer

Sloughy

Wet tissue

Absorb exudate

Treatment options

Larval therapy

Wet tissue

Control of exudate to ensure a balance between too much and too little presents practitioners with real clinical challenges. The aim of symptom control is to optimise exudate levels, protect the surrounding skin, and maximise the patient's quality of life by preventing leakage, controlling odour, and reducing pain (Cutting, 2004; Vowden and Vowden, 2004). Too much exudate can cause maceration and skin breakdown.

Treatment options ● Larval therapy

Larvae digest devitalised tissue by secreting proteolytic enzymes onto the wound bed, liquefying and breaking down dead tissue. Larvae ingest the liquefied tissue and other debris and bacteria.

In managing Phillip, the decision was made to use larval therapy. The rationale for doing so included:

❖ Application of a hydrogel or hydrocolloid dressing would be too moist, leading to maceration of the wound bed and surrounding skin.
❖ Too moist a wound environment might encourage bacterial growth and Phillip, due to his diabetes, was susceptible to infection.
❖ Larval therapy would provide rapid debridement. Again, due to his diabetes, the aim was to achieve a healthy wound bed, thus diminishing the risk of wound and systemic infection to which patients with diabetes are so vulnerable.

Evaluation of Phillip's care was undertaken and after three applications of larvae much of the sloughy tissue had been removed and a healthy wound bed remained. At this time the decision was made to stop the larval therapy and his wound care plan was changed accordingly.

Case scenario

Grace Pickard is a twenty-two-year-old clerical worker who, although in a steady relationship with her boyfriend, lives with her parents. Despite having spina bifida, Grace enjoys an active social life and works in a busy office environment. She has limited mobility and spends most of her waking hours in a wheelchair. Her wheelchair was commissioned and paid for by her parents to suit her body shape and lifestyle. She has a repositioning and moving plan to help ongoing pressure relief to pressure areas, but she sometimes forgets. Grace has had episodes of pressure ulceration to her feet, behind her knees, and to the sacral area. In the past, these have healed without complications. Following a Bank Holiday weekend, Grace notices drainage on her wheelchair cushion and an odour. She uses a mirror to inspect her perineal and sacral area and finds a discoloured area on her sacrum. Attending the GP's surgery as an emergency, an area of necrosis surrounded by inflamed, tender, oedematous tissue was noted. A provisional diagnosis of a grade 4 pressure ulcer with severe spreading infection was made. Grace's vital signs indicated that systemic infection was also present and she was admitted to hospital as an emergency for intravenous antibiotic therapy.

Grace's care plan reflected her deteriorating condition, focusing on control of her systemic infection and managing her pressure ulcer. Specifically, she required joint assessment by a surgeon and tissue viability nurse, relief of pressure with regular repositioning, monitoring of vital signs and ongoing monitoring of the pressure damage. It was important to determine whether immediate surgery was indicated, or whether it was safer to control the systemic and tissue infection prior to deciding on local wound care.

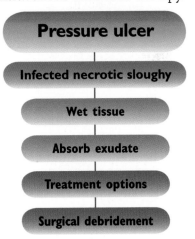

73

A joint review by the surgeon and tissue viability nurse, supported by a plain X-ray of the sacral area, led to a decision to treat Grace's systemic infection by intravenous antibiotics and to monitor her closely. Once her condition had settled, the plan was to debride the area surgically with a view to considering reconstructive plastic surgery in the future following complete resolution of infection. Wound assessment had identified a grade 4 pressure ulcer, comprising necrotic and sloughy tissue (*Figure 4.3*). There was a great deal of odour and signs of severe clinical infection. During this acute phase of Grace's illness, the wound symptoms were managed by using alginate dressings and absorbent padding.

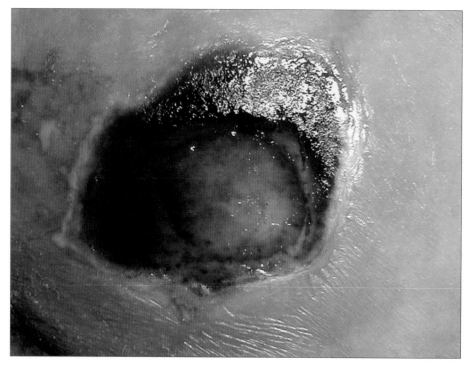

Figure 4.3: Grade 4 pressure ulcer with necrotic sloughy tissue

The rationale for doing so included:

❖ The alginate would absorb the large volumes of exudate that were produced by this pressure ulcer. Even though a cavity had not yet fully formed, tissue damage beneath the skin was extensive, producing copious exudate.

❖ The absorbent padding was used to supplement the alginate packing, as well as to facilitate regular inspection of the area. It was important that any rapid or further deterioration of the local tissue damage was detected so that immediate action could be taken.

❖ This regime allowed for the ongoing assessment of the spreading tissue infection surrounding the pressure ulcer.

Within five days Grace's physical condition had improved and her systemic infection resolved. After a further five days the local tissue infection had settled, but the wound continued to display signs of clinical infection. The priority of local wound care was now to debride the wound of necrotic and sloughy tissue.

The following pathway through the flow diagram was selected.

● **Treatment options** ● **Surgical debridement**

The decision was made to control the systemic and spreading tissue infection prior to performing surgical debridement. The rationale for doing so included:

❖ Grace was severely and acutely ill with a systemic infection and spreading tissue infection. The first priority was to stabilise her condition by using intravenous antibiotics.

❖ Once Grace's physical condition was stable, the next priority was to remove the necrotic and sloughy tissue in preparation for plastic surgery. The quickest way to achieve this was by surgical debridement in theatre by the surgeon.

Evaluation of Grace's care was undertaken after intravenous therapy had resolved the systemic and tissue infections. Following surgical debridement and creation of an acute wound, further evaluation confirmed that the wound bed was clean and free from infection, and her wound care plan was changed accordingly.

Pressure ulcer — granulating/epithelialising

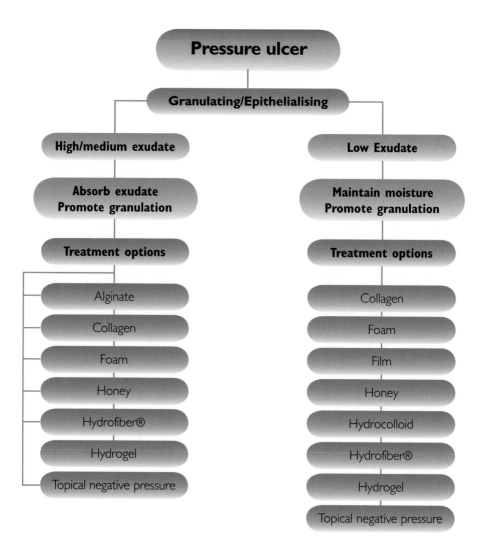

Case scenario

John Price is a seventy-two-year-old retired civil servant, widowed after fifty years of marriage, living by himself close to his daughter. He has gradually been coming to terms with the death of his wife and has started to play bowls and visit friends. John has been experiencing chest pain for some years and has been monitored for coronary heart disease, with a view to needing bypass surgery at some point. This stage was reached following several periods of severe chest pain that required admission to the coronary care unit. The surgical procedure was more complex than anticipated and John spent an extra five days in intensive care being stabilised. It was during this time that he developed a grade 3 pressure ulcer on his left elbow. John's general condition improved rapidly and he became mobile and independent. The care plan reflected his improved condition, focusing on rehabilitation and managing his pressure ulcer.

Specifically, he required relief of pressure to his elbow with a cushion and regular repositioning, ongoing physiotherapy, and monitoring of cardiac status. Wound assessment had identified a grade 3 pressure ulcer, mostly covered with healthy granulation tissue (*Figure 4.4*). There was no odour or clinical signs of infection. The priority of local wound care was to maintain a moist wound healing environment.

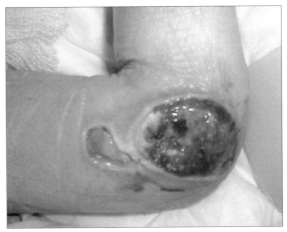

Figure 4.4: Grade 3 pressure ulcer to the elbow covered with granulation tissue

The following pathway through the flow diagram was selected.

● Granulating

Granulation tissue requires a moist environment so that exudate can bathe the wound bed. The beneficial properties of wound exudate have been demonstrated to promote healing in acute wounds (Parnham, 2002).

● Moist tissue

Control of exudate to ensure a balance between too much and too little is a key

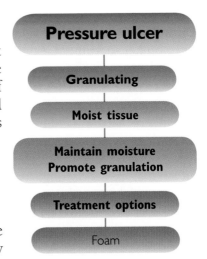

Pressure ulcer

Granulating

Moist tissue

Maintain moisture
Promote granulation

Treatment options

Foam

aim in optimising exudate levels. This also protects the surrounding skin and maximises the patient's quality of life by preventing leakage (Cutting, 2004; Vowden and Vowden, 2004).

● Treatment options ● Foam dressings

In managing John, the decision was made to use an adhesive foam dressing. The rationale for doing so included:

❖ In a healthy granulating wound bed, application of a foam dressing provides a moist environment conducive to healing.
❖ As the elbow is a difficult area in which to retain a dressing, an adhesive would hold the dressing in contact with the wound and would be advantageous over a non-adhesive foam dressing.

Evaluation of John's care was undertaken and the healthy granulating wound bed continued to heal.

Case scenario

Marion Conway is a seventy-nine-year-old retired dinner lady, widowed for eleven years, living by herself in a warden-controlled flat close to her daughter. She has had numerous minor illnesses throughout the winter and a chest infection that confined her to bed for more than two weeks. During this time she developed a small but painful grade 3 pressure ulcer on her sacrum. Marion's general condition slowly improved and she spent increasing amounts of time out of bed, getting around the flat. The district nurse visited Marion to assess and re-evaluate her dependence, as well as to manage her wound. The care plan reflected the frail and dependent nature of Marion's condition, focusing on rehabilitation and managing her pressure ulcer. Specifically, she required pressure-relieving equipment for her bed and chair, and encouragement and information on regular repositioning. Wound assessment had identified a grade 3 pressure ulcer, mostly covered with healthy epithelial tissue (*Figure 4.5*). There was no odour or clinical signs of infection. The priority of local wound care was to maintain a moist wound healing environment.

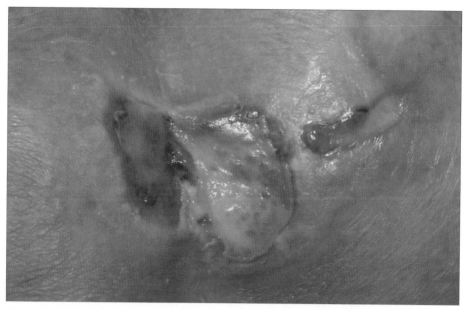

Figure 4.5: Grade 3 pressure ulcer to the sacrum with healthy, epithelial tissue

The following pathway through the flow diagram was selected.

Epithelialising

As wounds heal towards complete closure and produce little exudate, it is important to ensure that the wound bed does not dry out. Epithelial tissue requires a moist environment so that exudate can bathe the wound bed. A dry wound environment can inhibit the beneficial properties of wound exudate. Increased granulation tissue and wound contraction have been reported in a moist wound environment compared to a dry one (Parnham, 2002).

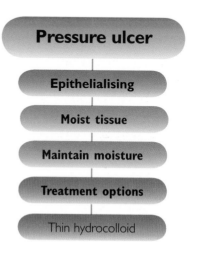

79

● Moist tissue

Control of exudate to ensure that moisture is retained in contact with the wound bed is a key aim in optimising epithelial growth and complete resurfacing of the wound bed.

● Treatment options ● Thin hydrocolloid dressings

In managing Marion, the decision was made to use a thin hydrocolloid dressing. The rationale for doing so included:

❖ Application of a hydrocolloid dressing would provide a moist environment conducive to healing in a healthy wound bed, progressing towards complete closure through epithelial growth.

❖ As Marion's skin is likely to be thin and fragile, an adhesive would hold the dressing in contact with the wound and would be advantageous over a non-adhesive dressing which would require surgical tape to secure the dressing which might cause skin damage and tears. These dressings are designed to stay in place for several days before a dressing change is needed, so the wound bed is not disturbed unnecessarily.

Traumatic wound

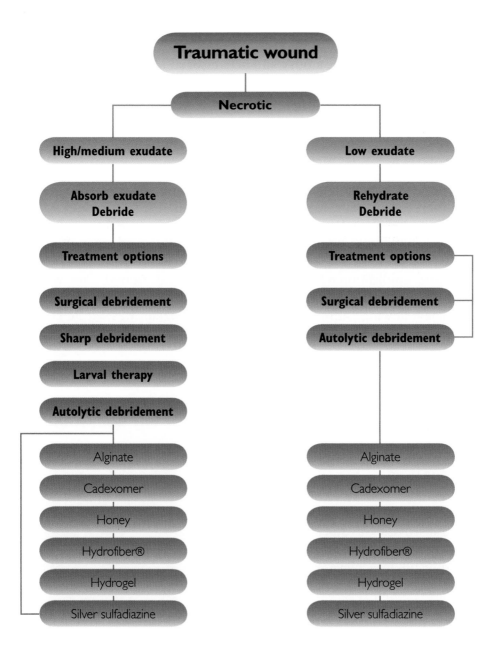

Case scenario

Michael Redwood is a thirty-year-old shop manager, married with two small children. He has a busy and active social life with his family. His wife usually drives their car, taking the children to school and then going on to work, so Michael takes his motorbike to the out of town sports shop where he is a manager. One wet day, the bike skidded and Michael fell off and scraped his arm on the tarmac. He was taken to hospital where a plain film X-ray confirmed that he had not broken any bones, but had a large, black, necrotic area on his upper arm. A nursing assessment highlighted that he was not covered for tetanus, required wound debridement and analgesia but, other than mild shock, was fit and healthy. Wound assessment identified a moderately exuding wound, filled with necrotic tissue. There was little odour, no clinical signs of infection, but Michael was experiencing procedural pain on dressing application. The first priority of local wound care was to debride the wound of necrotic tissue.

The following pathway through the flow diagram was selected.

● Necrotic

Necrosis comprises dead, non-viable tissue made up of dead cells, debris, fibrin and pus, providing an ideal medium to support bacterial growth (Schultz *et al*, 2004). To reduce the bioburden of the wound and to control or prevent infection, it is important to remove devitalised tissue as quickly and efficiently as possible (Ayello *et al*, 2004). This can be difficult to achieve as when necrotic tissue is firmly stuck to the wound bed it cannot simply be wiped away.

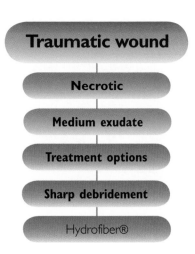

Medium exudate and necrotic tissue

❖ Moderate levels of exudate can be problematic as the wound bed can become macerated together with the surrounding skin, resulting in excoriation and an unhealthy wound bed.

❖ Exudate has a high content of protein, with cellular debris, bacteria and leukocytes that indicate health or the presence of disease (Baranoski and Ayello, 2004). Unhealthy exudate and wound environment is associated with inappropriate or defective cellular and cytokine activity (Hart, 2002; Moore, 1999; Park *et al*, 1998).

❖ Achieving the optimal level of exudate is a challenge as too much can cause maceration and skin breakdown (Cutting, 1999).

❖ When exposed to a moist environment, devitalised tissue undergoes a natural process of autolysis, where phagocytes and proteolytic enzymes soften and liquefy devitalised tissue, which is then digested by macrophages (Ayello *et al*, 2004).

Treatment options — Sharp debridement

Although Michael's wound is producing moderate levels of exudate and is likely over time to debride by the natural process of autolytic debridement, sharp debridement is an option that will accelerate this process by removing much of the devitalised tissue. This can be achieved in the A&E department with adequate pain control and involves:

❖ The devitalised or dead tissue is cut away from the healthy tissue by an experienced and competent practitioner who is knowledgeable about the anatomy of the area being debrided (Ayello *et al*, 2004).

❖ Thorough and effective surgical debridement down to healthy, viable tissue is best undertaken by a doctor with surgical skills or a specially trained nurse, as some bleeding usually results (Ramundo and Wells, 2000).

❖ In the UK, Fairbairn *et al* (2002) developed a framework for knowledge and competency-based practice to provide guidelines for nurses wishing to undertake sharp debridement. Application of a water-donating dressing, such as a hydrogel, is advised.

❖ Following this procedure, an absorbent dressing that prevents exudate from damaging the wound bed and surrounding skin can be applied, such as Hydrofiber®.

❖ Daily dressing changes would be undertaken initially, and then reviewed to ensure that the wound was left undisturbed as much as possible.

In managing Michael, the decision was made to undertake sharp debridement and then apply a Hydrofiber® dressing to absorb exudate, so protecting the wound bed and surrounding skin. The rationale for doing so included:

❖ Sharp debridement would quickly and effectively remove the devitalised tissue resulting in a healthier wound.
❖ Procedural pain would be reduced using analgesia prior to and following sharp debridement.
❖ The use of a Hydrofiber® dressing would help control exudate.
❖ Daily dressing changes were justified as the wound bed and surrounding skin should not become too macerated. Initially it was important for Michael to gain some experience from this dressing regime.

Evaluation of Michael's care was undertaken and, after the initial sharp debridement, much of the wound bed was healthy. However, moderate exudate levels meant that daily dressing changes were required to protect the wound bed and surrounding skin. Three days later, the exudate level started to decrease and dressing changes were required on alternate days. After a further five days, the wound bed was granulating and healthy and Michael's wound care plan was changed accordingly.

Traumatic wound — sloughy

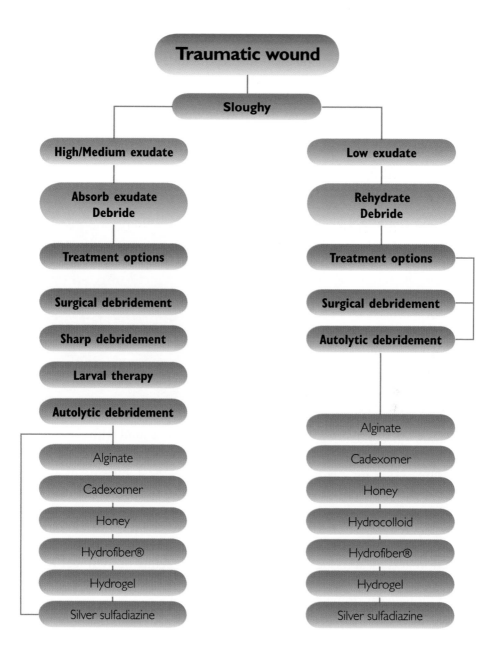

Case scenario

Margaret Barton is a seventy-six-year-old retired secretary, living alone in her own home. Her past medical history includes rheumatoid arthritis, for which she has required oral steroid medication for many years. This has left her with thin, papery skin that has only worsened as she has got older. Despite this, Margaret enjoys an active social life. She has fairly good mobility and takes public transport, walking short to moderate distances. Margaret has experienced minor skin tears to her forearms which, in the past, have healed without complication. Following a shopping trip to the supermarket on the bus, Grace notices that she has injured her shin and has a skin tear on her left shin that is oozing a small amount of blood. She applies a plaster, only to tear the skin further when she removes it following her evening bath. Attending the GP's surgery a few days later, the practice nurse notes that the skin surrounding the tear is extremely fragile, thin and papery, and is covered with sloughy tissue. At this time there are no clinical signs of infection present.

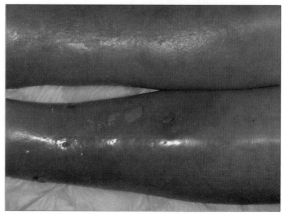

Figure 4.6: Traumatic wound with sloughy tissue

Margaret's care plan reflected her past medical history of taking steroids and the permanent damage that this has caused to her skin by focusing on maintaining the integrity of the remaining skin that is currently intact, while debriding the devitalised tissue from the wound bed. She also required monitoring for development of signs of clinical infection and local tissue infection. A dressing regime of hydrogel with a non-adherent dressing was selected. This was changed on alternate days. The rationale for doing so included:

❖ The hydrogel dressing would rehydrate the wound bed, facilitating autolysis.
❖ The non-adherent dressing would allow the dressings to be removed without further traumatising the wound area or the surrounding skin.

- ❖ Changing the dressing on alternate days would permit regular inspection of the area. It was important that any further deterioration of the local tissue damage was detected as soon as possible, as well as detecting the clinical signs of infection.
- ❖ This regime allowed for the ongoing assessment of the spreading tissue infection surrounding the wound, which might require more intensive intervention, such as the use of systemic antibiotics or even hospitalisation if a deep-seated tissue infection developed.

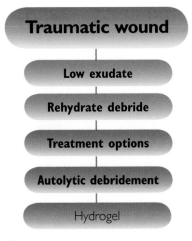

The following pathway through the flow diagram was selected.

● Treatment options ● Autolytic debridement

In managing Margaret, the decision was made to promote autolysis while protecting the skin surrounding the wound, rather than undertaking sharp or surgical debridement. The rationale for doing so included:

- ❖ Margaret was known to have thin, damaged, elderly and papery skin, which was extremely vulnerable to further damage and required protection. The first priority was to maintain the integrity of this skin and prevent further trauma.
- ❖ The next priority was to remove the sloughy tissue. The decision was made to promote autolysis using a water-based hydrogel dressing.

Within nine days Margaret's wound bed showed considerable progress towards debridement, with much of the devitalised tissue rehydrated and removed by the process of autolysis. Further evaluation confirmed that the wound bed was clean and free from infection and her wound care plan was changed accordingly.

Traumatic wound — granulating/epithelialising

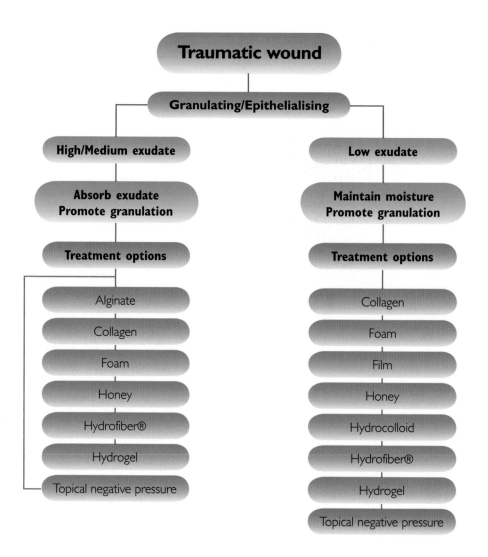

Case scenario

Jenny Probert is a fourteen-year-old school girl, living with her mother and younger brother. She is fit and healthy and enjoys a range of sporting activities, as well as socialising with her friends. While playing basketball for the school team, she slips over and gashes her leg on a nearby piece of gym equipment. The teacher takes Jenny to the local A&E for treatment. They wait for several hours and her mother arrives at the hospital. By the time Jenny is assessed, the wound is four hours old. The nurse assessing Jenny notes a small gash that has not been contaminated, but is too wide to suture. The priority of local wound care was to maintain a moist wound healing environment. A film dressing was selected for Jenny. This was changed when exudate gathered and leakage was imminent. The rationale for doing so included:

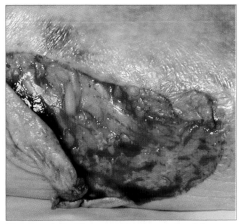

Figure 4.7: Traumatic wound with granulation and epithelial tissue

❖ In the presence of a healthy wound bed, promotion of granulation tissue would be facilitated by application of a film dressing that would provide a moist environment conducive to healing.
❖ Jenny would be able to bathe and shower as film dressings are semi-permeable. These dressings are designed to stay in place for several days before a dressing change is needed, so the wound bed would not be disturbed unnecessarily.

The following pathway through the flow diagram was selected.

Granulating

Granulation tissue requires a moist environment so that exudate can bathe the wound bed. The beneficial properties of wound exudate have been demonstrated to promote healing in acute wounds (Parnham, 2002). Increased numbers of macrophages, fibroblasts, myofibroblasts and increased granulation tissue and wound contraction were reported in a moist wound environment compared to a dry one.

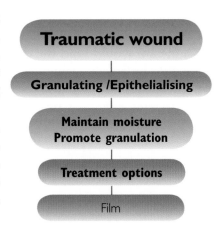

● Epithelialising

As wounds heal towards complete closure and produce little exudate, it is important to ensure that the wound bed does not dry out. Epithelial tissue requires a moist environment so that exudate can bathe the wound bed and new epithelial cells can migrate across the wound. Where there is superficial skin loss, remnants of hair follicles will act as sources of islands of epithelial cells that grow up out of the follicles. Migration of epithelial cells across the wound will continue until epithelial cells join up, covering the wound surface.

● Moist tissue

Control of exudate to ensure a balance between too much and too little is a key aim in optimising exudate level. This also protects the surrounding skin and maximises the patient's quality of life by preventing leakage (Cutting, 2004; Vowden and Vowden, 2004). Moisture, retained in contact with the wound bed, is a key aim in optimising epithelial growth and complete resurfacing of the wound bed.

● Treatment options ● Film dressings

In managing Jenny, the decision was made to use an adhesive film dressing. The rationale for doing so included:

❖ It would provide a moist environment conducive to healing.
❖ It would also be suitable for the wound once healthy granulation tissue was present.
❖ As the elbow is a difficult area in which to retain a dressing, an adhesive would hold the dressing in contact with the wound and would be advantageous over a non-adhesive foam dressing.
❖ These dressings are designed to stay in place for several days before a dressing change is needed, and so the wound bed would not be disturbed unnecessarily.

Evaluation of Jenny's care was undertaken and the healthy granulating wound bed was accompanied by the development of healthy epithelial tissue and the wound continued to heal.

Surgical wound — sloughy

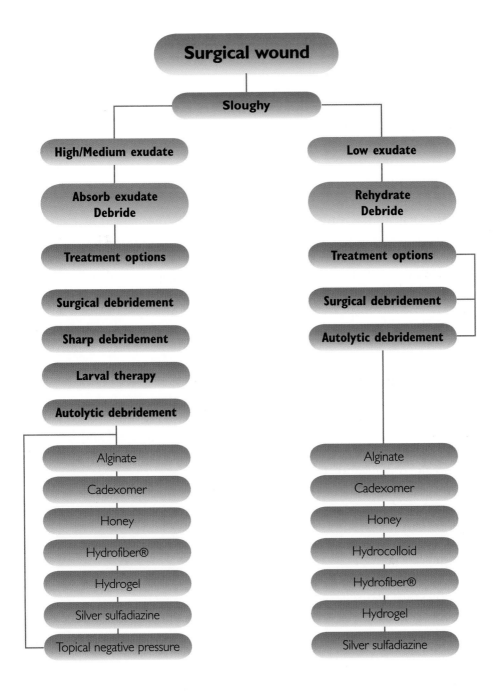

Case scenario

Simon Walters is a thirty-four-year-old bank clerk, living with his partner. Over the past four years, Simon has been aware of a small lump on his back, which was slowly but gradually getting larger. While swimming, his partner, John, noticed that this lump was larger than he remembered and he persuaded Simon to go to their GP to have the lump assessed. Both were anxious that it could be malignant. Following examination, the GP reassured Simon that this was a common condition, a lipoma. Simon was offered surgical excision due to the inconvenience that it was causing and the possibility of catching it and causing bleeding. Some six months later Simon was given an appointment for excision of lipoma in the ambulatory day unit. He attended and was discharged as expected on the same day. Enjoying a few days off from work on the advice of the surgeon, Simon decided to do some gardening, but slipped and pulled the wound open. He applied a sterile dressing pad that he had been given on his discharge home and hoped that it would heal quickly. Six days later John inspected the wound and found a sloughy, dry wound bed, which Simon was finding increasingly uncomfortable. They visited their GP the next day, who referred them to the practice nurse for assessment and treatment. She assessed Simon's wound, establishing that he was otherwise healthy with no clinical signs of infection locally, and no deeper tissue infection in the surrounding skin. Wound assessment identified a sloughy wound that was largely dry.

The first priority of local wound care was to rehydrate and facilitate autolytic debridement of sloughy tissue. Wounds on the back are prone to break down and become infected because of the thickness of the skin in this area, and a less prolific blood supply than other parts of the body. A treatment to reduce the bacterial load would benefit Simon.

The following pathway through the flow diagram was selected.

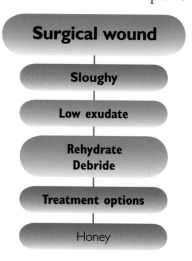

● Sloughy

Slough comprises dead, non-viable tissue made up of dead cells, debris, fibrin and pus, providing an ideal medium to support bacterial growth (Schultz _et al_, 2004). It is important to remove devitalised tissue as quickly and efficiently as possible to reduce the bioburden of the wound and to control or prevent infection (Ayello _et al_, 2004). This can be difficult to achieve as sloughy tissue is firmly stuck to the wound bed and it cannot simply be wiped away.

Dry tissue

Too little wound exudate can also be problematic as the wound bed dries out, leaving a scab or layer of dessicated exudate. Research has demonstrated that healing is delayed in a dry wound environment in both an animal model (Winter, 1962) and in human skin (Hinman and Maibach, 1963; Eaglestein, 1985). With sloughy tissue, the devitalised tissue has died and formed a firm covering. A dry wound environment can inhibit the beneficial properties of wound exudate. Increased granulation tissue and wound contraction were reported in a moist wound environment compared to a dry one (Parnham, 2002).

Rehydrate and debride

When exposed to a moist environment, devitalised tissue undergoes a natural process of autolysis where phagocytes and proteolytic enzymes soften and liquefy devitalised tissue, which is then digested by macrophages (Ayello _et al_, 2004).

Treatment options Honey

❖ Dressings that reduce the bacterial load include antiseptics and honey, which provide a moist wound environment that facilitates autolysis.

In managing Simon's wound, the decision was made to apply a honey dressing and hold this in place with a semi-permeable film dressing, initially changed on alternate days. The rationale for doing so included:

❖ The activity of a honey dressing would facilitate autolytic debridement (White and Molan, 2005).

❖ It would also provide the moist wound environment needed to encourage the natural process of autolytic debridement.

❖ It would reduce the bacterial load on the wound bed through antimicrobial activity (Cooper, 2005).

❖ The use of a semi-permeable film dressing would help to protect the wound from further contamination.

❖ Alternate day dressing changes were justified as the wound bed would not dry out and regular inspection was needed to detect the clinical signs of infection.

Evaluation of Simon's care was undertaken and, after fifteen days, all of the sloughy tissue had been rehydrated and had separated from the wound bed, leaving it healthy and granulating. The wound care plan was modified accordingly.

Although honey has been used for millennia, only in recent years has the mode of action been explored and a therapeutic concentration developed. Molan (2005) describes a variety of bioactivities of honey, including debridement, inflammation suppression, bacteriocidal activity, and stimulation of healing. With respect to debridement, honey is thought to have several effects, namely:

• acceleration of autolytic debridement, possibly through the activation of proteases that digest devitalised tissue (Subrahmanyam, 1996)
• effective penetration of hard eschar (Molan, 2005)
• conversion of inactive plasminogen to active plasmin, which breaks down fibrin clots that attach slough and eschar to the wound bed (Esmon, 2004)
• osmotic activity that draws in water to wash the surface of the wound, removing debris (Molan, 2002).

Surgical wound — granulating/epithelialising

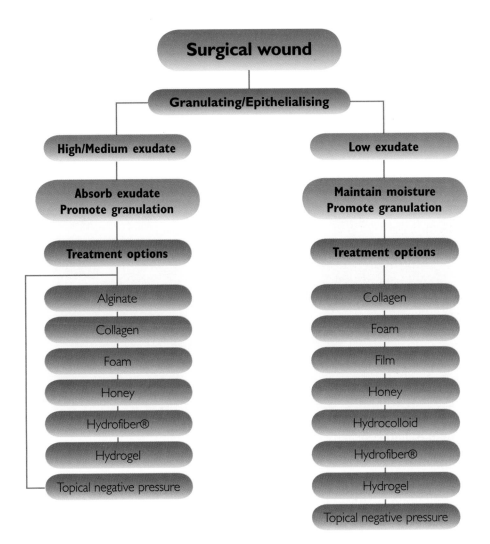

Case scenario

Bill Draper is a fifty-seven-year-old builder, living with his wife. He was fit and active and had his own building business. He developed severe abdominal pain and was admitted as an emergency, diagnosed with bowel obstruction and immediately operated on. He had faecal peritonitis from a ruptured bowel as a result of colonic cancer, which required surgery to remove the cancer and repair the ruptured bowel. Due to the gross contamination of the abdominal cavity, his abdominal wound was left open to drain and heal by secondary intention. A large, heavily exuding cavity wound resulted (*Figure 4.8*). The priority of local wound care was to control the large amount of exudate, so that the wound bed and surrounding skin would not be damaged and excoriated. Treatment with topical negative pressure (TNP) was selected for Bill. The rationale for doing so included:

❖ In the presence of such a large volume of exudate, cavity dressings would not be able to absorb sufficient exudate, anticipating frequent dressing changes.
❖ Such a large wound would benefit from the stimulation of granulation tissue that the TNP therapy promotes.

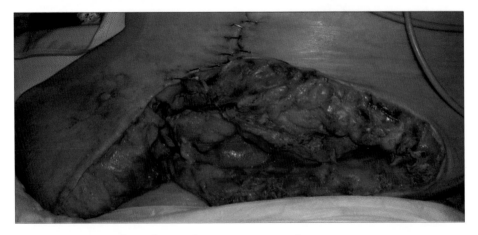

Figure 4.8: Large, heavily exuding cavity wound

The following pathway through the flow diagram was selected.

● Granulating

Granulation tissue requires a moist environment so that exudate can bathe the wound bed. The beneficial properties of wound exudate have been demonstrated to promote healing in acute wounds (Parnham, 2002). Increased numbers of macrophages, fibroblasts, myofibroblasts and increased granulation tissue and wound contraction were reported in a moist wound environment compared to a dry one.

Moist tissue

Control of exudate, ensuring a balance between too much and too little, is a key aim in optimising exudate levels (Cutting, 2004; Vowden and Vowden, 2004). Excess moisture is also absorbed to reduce the possibility of maceration to the wound bed and surrounding skin.

Surgical wound

Granulating/Epithelialising

High/Medium exudate

Absorb exudate
Promote granulation

Treatment options

TNP

Treatment options ● Topical negative pressure therapy

In managing Bill, the decision was made to use TNP therapy. The rationale for doing so included:

❖ It would absorb excess exudate, so preventing maceration.
❖ It would also promote granulation tissue production and so enhance or accelerate healing.

Evaluation of Bill's care was undertaken and the healthy granulating wound bed was achieved with TNP therapy. Once the exudate level had reduced sufficiently for cavity wound dressings to be managed, this treatment was discontinued.

Topical negative pressure applies sub-atmospheric, negative pressure to the wound bed via a computerised device (Baranoski and Ayello, 2004). A sponge dressing is applied to the wound bed and sealed using an adhesive film dressing, which is connected to the suction device, removing excess fluid from the wound bed. It is thought that negative pressure also stimulates granulation tissue formation and reduces bacterial counts (Broussard et al, 2000). In some cases, granulation tissue has formed over exposed bone and implants. Other benefits include increased local blood perfusion, increased nutrient delivery to wounded tissue, and accelerated rate of granulation tissue.

Surgical wound — necrotic

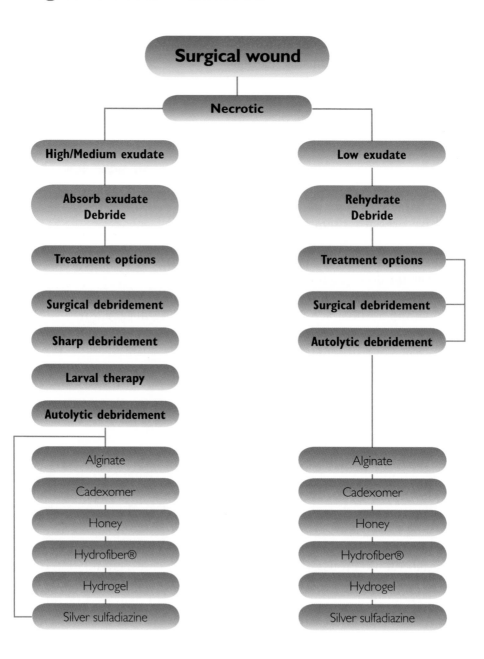

Case scenario

Polly Tucker is a forty-seven-year-old librarian, single and living with her sister Dawn on a smallholding just outside their town. Discovering a lump in her breast, Polly goes to her GP and is fast-tracked through the local breast care centre. She is diagnosed with breast cancer and elects to have mastectomy with immediate reconstruction. The operation is successful, though four days post-operatively a large section of skin on the edge of the reconstructed breast begins to turn a dusky colour and gradually becomes necrotic (*Figure 4.9*). The surgeon and Polly decide that surgical excision is the best option to get the problem resolved quickly. There was little odour and no clinical signs of infection. The first priority of local wound care was to debride the wound of necrotic tissue.

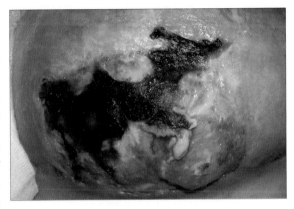

Figure 4.9: Surgical necrotic wound

The following pathway through the flow diagram was selected.

● Necrotic

Necrosis comprises dead, non-viable tissue, made up of dead cells, debris, fibrin and pus, providing an ideal medium to support bacterial growth (Schultz *et al*, 2004). It is important to remove devitalised tissue as quickly and efficiently as possible to reduce the bioburden of the wound and to control or prevent infection (Ayello *et al*, 2004). This can be difficult to achieve as when necrotic tissue is firmly stuck to the wound bed it cannot simply be wiped away.

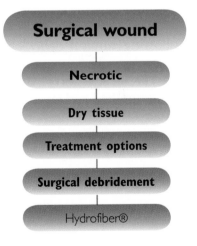

Treatment options • Surgical debridement

Although Polly's wound is dry and not producing high levels of exudate, it is likely that, due to the extensive amount of tissue lost, the area will become moist and leak moderate to large amounts of malodorous fluid as the natural autolytic processes take place. Surgical debridement by the surgeon in theatre will remove the devitalised tissue in one surgical procedure and result in a healthy wound bed. Following this procedure, a dressing that absorbs exudate and prevents excessive amounts from damaging the wound bed and surrounding skin can be applied, such as Hydrofiber®.

Initially, dressing changes would take place on alternate days, but this would be reviewed to ensure that the wound was left as undisturbed as possible.

In managing Polly, the decision was made to undertake surgical debridement and then apply a Hydrofiber® dressing to absorb exudate, so protecting the wound bed and surrounding skin. The rationale for doing so included:

❖ Surgical debridement undertaken by a surgeon quickly and effectively removes the devitalised tissue, resulting in a healthy wound.
❖ Undertaking this procedure in theatre is the only feasible way to reduce the likelihood of pain.
❖ The use of a Hydrofiber® dressing would help control exudate.
❖ Dressing changes on alternate days were justified as the wound bed and surrounding skin should not become too macerated. These would be reduced as the levels of exudate decreased.

Following surgical debridement, further evaluation of Polly's care was undertaken. The wound bed was now healthy but moderate exudate levels meant that fairly frequent dressing changes were required to protect the wound bed and surrounding skin. Seven days later, the exudate level started to decrease and dressing changes were required every three days. After a further five days, the wound bed was granulating and healthy and Polly's wound care plan was changed accordingly.

Leg ulcer — granulating/epithelialising

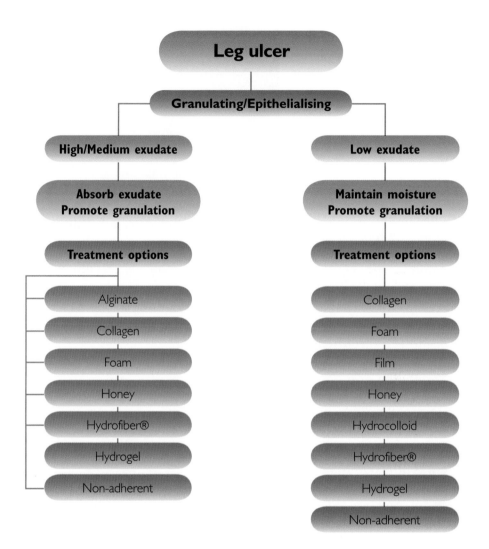

Case scenario

Josie King is a sixty-four-year-old retired flight attendant, married and living with her husband. They have a busy life travelling to visit the many friends that they made while Josie worked for the airline industry. Josie has had severe varicose veins for many years and has experienced two previous episodes of venous leg ulceration. These have been successfully treated using four-layer bandages. Two months ago she developed another ulcer close to the medial malleolus. Returning to her practice nurse, an assessment was carried out based on NICE Guidelines (NICE, 2001). The outcomes were:

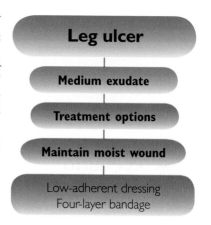

Figure 4.10: Granulating epithelialising leg ulcer

❖ History taking — severe venous disease with previous episodes of ulceration.
❖ Examination of the skin condition surrounding the wound — dry, ezematous, oedematous skin and wound assessment.
❖ Investigation — ankle brachial pressure index (ABPI) to detect vascular insufficiency with a result of an index of 0.95.
❖ Diagnosis — recurrence of venous ulceration.
❖ Intervention — compression bandages, emollients to surrounding skin.

Wound assessment identified a moderately exuding ulcer, filled with healthy tissue and with an epithelialising wound edge. There was little odour, no clinical signs of infection and little discomfort. The first priority of care was to apply sustained compression.

The following pathway through the flow diagram was selected.

Leg ulcer

Medium exudate

Treatment options

Maintain moist wound

Low-adherent dressing
Four-layer bandage

● **Moist tissue**

Control of exudate, ensuring a balance between too much and too little, is a key aim in optimising exudate levels (Cutting, 2004; Vowden and Vowden, 2004). It also ensures that excess moisture is absorbed to reduce the possibility of maceration to the wound bed and surrounding skin.

● Granulating

Granulation tissue requires a moist environment so that exudate can bathe the wound bed. A dry wound environment can inhibit the beneficial properties of wound exudate. Increased granulation tissue and wound contraction were reported in a moist wound environment compared to a dry one (Parnham, 2002).

● Epithelialising

As wounds heal towards complete closure and produce little exudate, it is important to ensure that the wound bed does not dry out. Epithelial tissue requires a moist environment so that exudate can bathe the wound bed. A dry wound environment can inhibit the beneficial properties of wound exudate, which has been demonstrated to promote healing by increasing numbers of macrophages, fibroblasts, and myofibroblasts. Increased granulation tissue and wound contraction were reported in a moist wound environment compared to a dry one (Parnham, 2002).

● Treatment options ● Low-adherent dressing and compression bandaging

In managing Josie, the decision was made to use a low-adherent dressing. The rationale for doing so included:

❖ Used in conjunction with compression bandaging, this would provide a moist environment conducive to healing.
❖ These dressings are designed to stay in place for several days before a dressing change is needed, and so would be suitable for use with the four-layer bandages that could stay in place for a week.

Evaluation of Josie's care was undertaken every week when the bandages were changed. The ulcer healed after eleven weeks and she was fitted and supplied with compression hosiery (Best Practice Statement, Compression Hosiery, 2005, available online from: www.wounds-uk.com).

Leg ulcer — sloughy

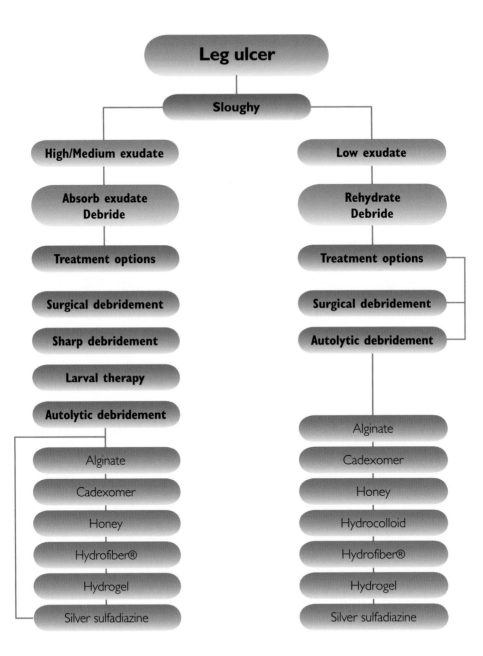

Case scenario

John Sutton is a sixty-nine-year-old retired engineer, living alone in his own home. His past medical history includes mild peripheral vascular disease. John lives a quiet life. He has fairly good mobility and takes public transport, walking short to moderate distances. John knocked his leg while gardening, and over the following four weeks noticed a gradual enlarging of the wound. His son became worried as the wound deteriorated and took John to the local GP's surgery the next day. The practice nurse performed an assessment based on NICE Guidelines (NICE, 2001). The outcomes were:

❖ History taking — mixed venous and arterial disease with no previous episodes of ulceration.
❖ Examination of the skin condition surrounding the wound — dry, oedematous skin with no evidence of tissue infection, and wound assessment.
❖ Investigation — ABPI to detect vascular insufficiency with a result of an index of 0.65.
❖ Diagnosis — mixed disease.
❖ Intervention — topical antimicrobial dressings, light compression bandages, emollients to surrounding skin.

Wound assessment identified a moderately exuding ulcer, covered with sloughy tissue (_Figure 4.11_). There was little odour, no clinical signs of infection and little discomfort. The first priority of care was to debride the sloughy tissue, as this could be a focus for bacterial growth that might result in infection.

The following pathway through the flow diagram was selected.

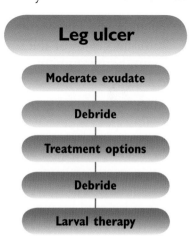

● Slough

Slough comprises dead, non-viable tissue made up of dead cells, debris, fibrin and pus, providing an ideal medium to support bacterial growth (Schultz _et_ *al*, 2004). It is important to remove devitalised tissue as quickly and efficiently as possible (Ayello *et al*, 2004).

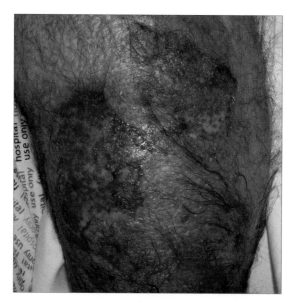

Figure 4.11: Leg ulcer with sloughy tissue

● Moderate exudate and necrotic tissue

❖ Moderate levels of exudate can be problematic as the wound bed can become macerated together with the surrounding skin, resulting in excoriation and an unhealthy wound bed.

❖ Exudate has a high content of protein, with cellular debris, bacteria and leukocytes (Baranoski and Ayello, 2004), which indicate health or the presence of disease. Unhealthy exudate and wound environment is associated with inappropriate or defective cellular and cytokine activity (Hart, 2002; Moore, 1999; Park *et al*, 1998).

❖ Achieving the optimal level of exudate is a challenge as too much exudate can cause maceration and skin breakdown (Cutting, 1999).

❖ When exposed to a moist environment, devitalised tissue undergoes a natural process of autolysis where phagocytes and proteolytic enzymes soften and liquefy devitalised tissue, which is then digested by macrophages (Ayello *et al*, 2004).

● Treatment options ● Larval therapy

Larvae digest devitalised tissue by secreting proteolytic enzymes onto the wound bed, liquefying and breaking down dead tissue. Larvae ingest the liquefied tissue and other debris and bacteria. In managing John, the decision was made to use larval therapy. The rationale for doing so included:

❖ Application of a hydrogel or hydrocolloid dressing would be too moist, leading to maceration of the wound bed and surrounding skin.
❖ Too moist a wound environment might encourage bacterial growth and, in the presence of vascular disease, John was susceptible to infection.
❖ Larval therapy would provide rapid debridement. Again, due to his vascular impairment, the aim was to achieve a healthy wound bed, diminishing the risk of wound and systemic infection that patients with vascular disease are vulnerable to developing.

Evaluation of John's care was undertaken and after two applications of larvae much of the sloughy tissue had been removed and a healthy wound bed remained. At this time the decision was made to stop the larval therapy and his wound care plan was changed accordingly.

Leg ulcer — necrotic

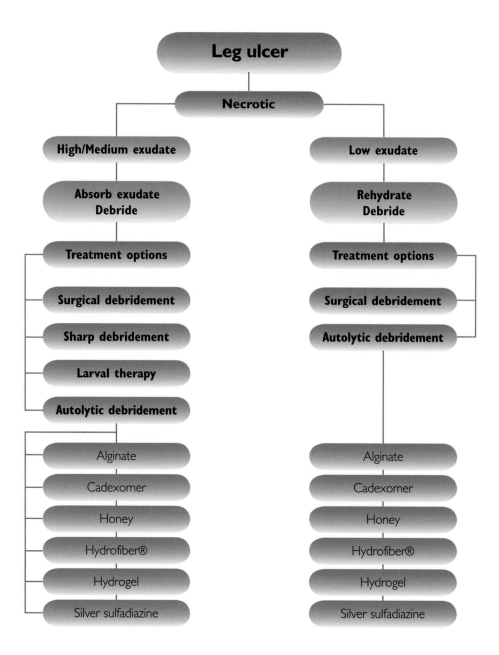

Case scenario

Milly Wright is a seventy-eight-year-old housewife, living with her younger sister in their own home. She is quite frail and rarely goes out, but enjoys pottering in the garden, as well as receiving visits from her friends. Milly has noticed that her feet are cold even in the summer, and she also has intermittent pain in her lower legs. She scraped her leg on a rose bush and the cut became ulcerated and painful. Following a telephone call to the GP's surgery, arrangements were made for the district nurse to call and assess Milly. She assessed Milly using NICE Guidelines (NICE, 2001). The outcomes were:

❖ History taking — no previous episodes of ulceration, but pain in the lower leg and cold feet.
❖ Examination of the skin condition surrounding the wound — a cold, poorly perfused foot with no evidence of tissue infection. Wound assessment revealed a necrotic wound bed, oozing heavily.
❖ Investigation — ABPI to detect vascular insufficiency with a result of an index of 0.45. Referral to a vascular surgeon for further investigation and advice.
❖ Provisional diagnosis — ischaemic, arterial ulceration.
❖ Intervention — silver alginate dressings held in place with light retention bandages.

Wound assessment identified a heavily exuding ulcer, covered with necrotic tissue (_Figure 4.12_). There was some malodour, no clinical signs of infection, and a little discomfort. The first priority of care was to debride the necrotic tissue while waiting for a vascular opinion.

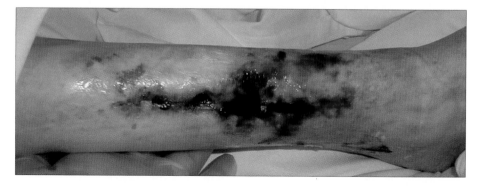

Figure 4.12: Leg ulcer, necrotic

The following pathway through the flow diagram was selected.

● Necrotic

Necrosis comprises dead, non-viable tissue made up of dead cells, debris, fibrin and pus, providing an ideal medium to support bacterial growth (Schultz *et al*, 2004). It is important to remove devitalised tissue as quickly and efficiently as possible to reduce the bioburden of the wound and to control or prevent infection (Ayello *et al*, 2004). This can be difficult to achieve as when necrotic tissue is firmly stuck to the wound bed it cannot simply be wiped away.

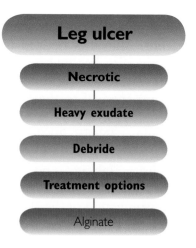

● Heavy exudate and necrotic tissue

❖ High levels of exudate can be problematic as the wound bed, together with the surrounding skin, can become macerated, resulting in excoriation and an unhealthy wound bed.
❖ Exudate has a high content of protein, with cellular debris, bacteria and leukocytes (Baranoski and Ayello, 2004), indicating health or the presence of disease. Unhealthy exudate and wound environment are associated with inappropriate or defective cellular and cytokine activity (Hart, 2002; Moore, 1999; Park *et al*, 1998).
❖ Achieving the optimal level of exudate is a challenge as too much exudate can cause maceration and skin breakdown (Cutting, 1999).

● Treatment options ● Alginate dressing

In managing Milly's wound, the decision was made to apply a silver alginate dressing and hold this in place with absorbent padding and a light retention bandage, initially changed every day. The rationale for this included:

❖ Silver contained in the alginate dressing would absorb exudate while reducing the bacterial load on the wound bed.

❖ It would also provide some moisture needed to encourage the natural process of autolytic debridement.

❖ The use of absorbent padding would help absorb excess exudate and protect the surrounding skin from maceration.

❖ Daily dressing changes were justified on the grounds that the exudate was heavy initially, and frequent wound inspection was needed to detect the clinical signs of infection locally in the wound, and also in the surrounding tissues.

Evaluation of Milly's care was undertaken and after eleven days the exudate had reduced and much of the necrotic tissue had separated from the wound bed, leaving patches of healthier granulation tissue. The wound care plan was then modified accordingly.

Diabetic foot — necrotic/sloughy

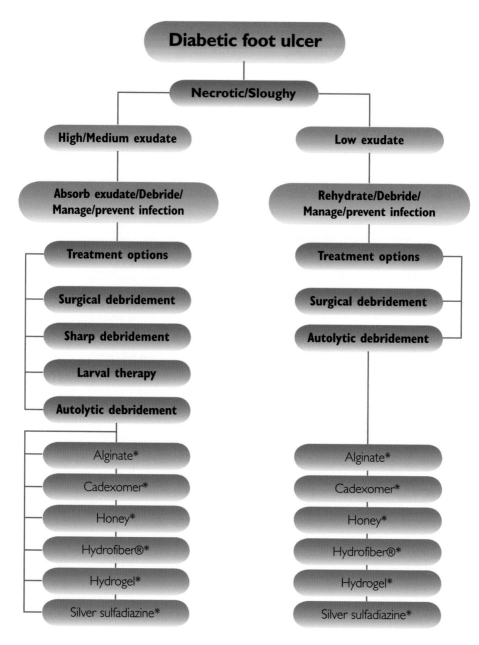

* Some of the products in these categories contain antimicrobials suitable for the management/prevention of infection

Case scenario

Vijay Singh is a seventy-two-year-old retired pharmacist, widowed for nine years and living with his daughter and her family. Diagnosed with diabetes in his forties, Vijay has managed to gain good control over his diabetes, but as the disease has progressed he has been insulin dependent for twelve years. He is meticulous with respect to monitoring his blood glucose levels but, despite this, has experienced several episodes of foot ulceration over the past fifteen years. The local district general hospital have a multi-professional diabetic foot clinic, where Vijay attends for annual screening when he is ulcer free, and for treatment at the times when his foot becomes ulcerated. Nine months ago another foot ulcer appeared, and this time a foot assessment detected significant ischaemic disease in his lower leg. The staff at the diabetic foot clinic have been carefully monitoring his progress.

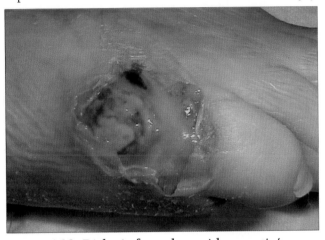

Figure 4.13: Diabetic foot ulcer with necrotic/ sloughy tissue

Standard assessment and management at this clinic are based on NICE Guidelines (NICE, 2004) which includes:

❖ **_Lower limb assessment._** Examination in the clinical setting is a fundamental step to identifying risk factors in the foot to reduce risk of ulceration and amputation (Mayfield *et al*, 1998). This examination takes a short period of time and healthcare professionals need to realise how important the detection and monitoring of neuropathy and foot complications are (Boulton, 1995). Neurological assessment can be carried out using simple practical tests to define loss of vibration and protective sensations. Assessment requires careful history taking, clinical examination and avoiding the reliance on a single finding (Fowler and Mitchell, 1998). This includes foot colour, skin temperature, callus build, hair loss on the dorsum (Mayfield *et al*, 1998; Santos and Carline, 2000).

❖ **Management of foot ulceration.** The minimal standard care of foot ulceration includes:

- *Regular removal of callus:* callus can lead to increased pressure in the tissues and rupturing of blood capillaries (Bale and Harding, 2000). Callus build up can also delay epithelial migration from the ulcer edge.
- *Offloading pressure:* orthotic devices such as specialised shoes, braces and boots, total contact casting (Edmonds and Foster, 2000).
- *Antimicrobial dressings:* these can help reduce bacterial growth, so helping to prevent infection.
- *Control of diabetes:* To reduce the chances of infection.
- *Frequent inspection for the early detection of infection:* this is essential as localised infection can rapidly spread to the surrounding tissues, leading to deterioration in the limb, gangrene and amputation. This is particularly relevant when ischaemia is known to be present, as in Vijay's case.

The following pathway through the flow diagram was selected.

● Slough

Slough comprises dead, non-viable tissue consisting of dead cells, debris, fibrin and pus, which provides an ideal medium to support bacterial growth (Schutlz *et al*, 2004). It is important to remove devitalised tissue as quickly and efficiently as possible to reduce the bioburden of the wound and to control or prevent infection (Ayello *et al*, 2004). This can be difficult as when necrotic tissue is firmly stuck to the wound bed it cannot simply be wiped away. For patients with diabetes, infection can

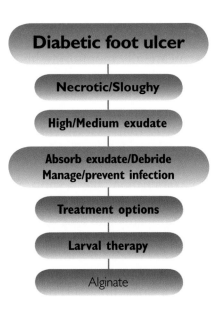

Diabetic foot ulcer

Necrotic/Sloughy

High/Medium exudate

Absorb exudate/Debride
Manage/prevent infection

Treatment options

Larval therapy

Alginate

have devastating consequences if it is not quickly resolved, resulting in amputation or, in extreme cases, death.

Debride

When exposed to a moist environment, devitalised tissue undergoes a natural process of autolysis, where phagocytes and proteolytic enzymes soften and liquefy devitalised tissue, which is then digested by macrophages.

Treatment options ● Larval therapy

Larvae digest devitalised tissue by secreting proteolytic enzymes onto the wound bed, liquefying and breaking down dead tissue. Larvae ingest the liquefied tissue and other debris and bacteria.

In managing Vijay, the decision was made to use larval therapy. The rationale for doing so included:

❖ Application of a hydrogel or hydrocolloid dressing would be too moist and lead to maceration of the wound bed and surrounding skin.
❖ Too moist a wound environment might encourage bacterial growth and, due to his diabetes, Vijay was very susceptible to infection.
❖ Larval therapy would provide rapid debridement. Again, due to his diabetes, the aim was to achieve a healthy wound bed, diminishing the risk of wound and systemic infection to which patients with diabetes are so vulnerable.

Evaluation of Vijay's care was undertaken and after four applications of larvae much of the sloughy tissue had been removed and a healthy wound bed remained. At this time, the decision was made to stop the larval therapy and his wound care plan was changed accordingly.

In addition, ongoing care was given by the diabetic foot clinic. The rationale for doing so included:

❖ Patients cared for by a multi-professional diabetic foot team have improved outcomes (Edmonds and Foster, 2000; Plank _et al_, 2003).
❖ Patients that are managed by diabetic foot teams experience reduced rates of complications, especially infection and amputation (Armstrong _et al_, 1999).

Evaluation of Vijay's care was undertaken and, after two weeks, much of the necrotic tissue had been digested from the wound bed and the clinical signs of infection remained absent. At this time the decision was made to change to a silver alginate dressing to help reduce the bacterial load.

Diabetic foot ulcer — granulating/epithelialising

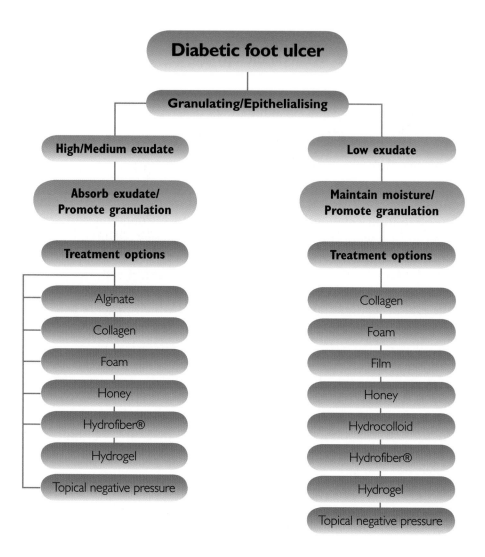

Case scenario

Patrick Michaels is a fifty-seven-year-old travel agent, living with his wife and youngest daughter. He developed late-onset diabetes ten years ago and, over this time, has experienced difficulties in sticking to a diet different from his previous diet and in controlling his diabetes. His work involves socialising at lunchtimes and eating business lunches consisting of fatty and sugary foods. This has resulted in high and unstable blood sugar values when he finds the time to test his levels. Patrick doesn't often attend the diabetic foot clinic and regularly misses his annual reviews. He doesn't like wearing orthotic shoes and rarely inspects his feet for damage. He has limited support from his wife, who enjoys going out with her husband in the evenings to their local pub.

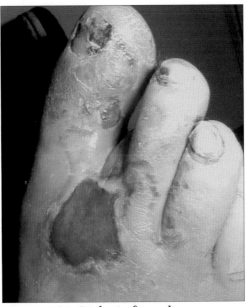

Just before going on holiday Patrick buys a new pair of shoes. Not knowing that he now has neuropathy, he fails to realise that these shoes are ill-fitting and rub the dorsum aspect of one foot. On returning from holiday his wife notices that his socks are stained and, on inspection, Patrick finds a reddened area with an open weeping ulcer (_Figure 4.14_). He finds the telephone number of

Figure 4.14: Diabetic foot ulcer, granulating and epithelialising

the diabetic foot clinic and manages to get an appointment for that day. A full lower limb assessment is performed based on NICE Guidelines, including:

- a neurological assessment
- history taking
- clinical examination (foot colour, skin temperature, callus build, hair loss on the dorsum of the foot).

A diagnosis is made of traumatic foot ulceration as a result of an insensate foot, with no infection and a healthy ulcer measuring 1 x 1.5 cm.

The following pathway through the flow diagram was selected.

Granulating

Granulation tissue requires a moist environment so that exudate can bathe the wound bed. A dry wound environment can inhibit the beneficial properties of wound exudate, which has been demonstrated to promote healing by increasing numbers of macrophages, fibroblasts, and myofibroblasts. Increased granulation tissue and wound contraction were reported in a moist wound environment compared to a dry one (Parnham, 2002).

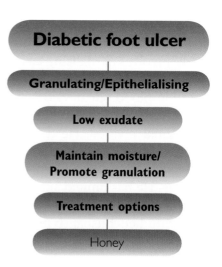

Epithelialising

As wounds heal towards complete closure and produce little exudate, it is important to ensure that the wound bed does not dry out. Epithelial tissue requires a moist environment so that exudate can bathe the wound bed. A dry wound environment can inhibit the beneficial properties of wound exudate, which has been demonstrated to promote healing by increasing numbers of macrophages, fibroblasts, and myofibroblasts. Increased granulation tissue and wound contraction were reported in a moist wound environment compared to a dry one (Parnham, 2002). .

Moist tissue

Control of exudate, to ensure a balance between too much and too little, is a key aim in optimising exudate levels. This also protects the surrounding skin and maximises the patient's quality of life by preventing leakage (Cutting, 2004; Vowden and Vowden, 2004).

Treatment options Honey

In managing Simon's wound, the decision was made to apply a honey dressing held in place with a low-adherent dressing, initially changed on alternate days. The rationale for doing so included:

* It would provide a moist wound environment needed to encourage the natural process of autolytic debridement.
* It would reduce the bacterial load on the wound bed through antimicrobial activity (Cooper, 2005).
* The use of a low-adherent dressing would help to keep the dressing in place and keep the honey in contact with the wound bed
* Alternate day dressing changes ensured that the wound bed did not dry out and gave the opportunity for regular inspection.

Evaluation of Patrick's care was undertaken and the healthy granulating wound bed continued to heal.

Conclusion

This chapter has illustrated how the flow diagrams can be used in clinical practice by presenting a series of patient case scenarios. These are examples of patients that could form the practice of nurses in their everyday working environment. Be encouraged to use them as part of taking a structured and logical approach when caring for your patients.

References

Ayello AE, Baranoski S, Kerstein MD, Cuddigan J (2004) Wound debridement. In: _Wound Care Essentials: Practice principles._ Lippincott Williams & Wilkins, Philadelphia

Bale S, Harding K (2000) Chronic wounds 2: Diabetic foot ulcers and malignant wounds. In: Bale S, Harding K, Leaper , eds. _An Introduction to Wounds._ EMAP Healthcare Ltd, London

Baranoski S, Ayello EA (2004) Wound treatment options. In: Baranoski S, Ayello EA, eds. *Wound Care Essentials: Practice principles*. Lippincott Williams and Wilkins, Philadelphia

Boulton AJM (1996) The diabetic foot. *Surgery* **14**(2): 37–9

Broussard GL, Mendez-Eastman S, Frantz R (2000) Adjuvant wound therapies. In: Bryant RA, ed. *Acute & Chronic Wounds: Nursing Management*. Mosby, St Louis

Cutting KF (2004) Wound exudate: composition and functions. In: White R, ed. *Trends in Wound Care, volume III*. Quay Books, MA Healthcare Ltd, London

Edmonds ME, Foster AVM (2000) *Managing the Diabetic Foot*. Blackwells, Oxford

Eaglestein WH (1985) Experiences with biosythetic dressings. *J Am Acad Dermatol* **12**: 434–40

Esmon CT (2004) Crosstalk between inflammation and thrombosis. *Maturas* **47**(4): 305–14

Fairbairn K, Grier J, Hunter C, Preece J (2002) A sharp debridement procedure devised by specialist nurses. *J Wound Care* **11**(10): 371–5

Hinman CD, Maibach HI (1963) Effect of air exposure and occlusion on experimental human skin wounds. *Nature* **200**: 377

Mayfield JA, Reiber GE, Sanders LJ, Janisse D, Pogach LM (1998) Preventative foot care in people with diabetes. *Diabetes Care* **21**(12): 2161–86

Molan P (2002) Re-introducing honey in the management of wounds and ulcers — theory and practice. *Ostomy/Wound Management* **48**(11): 28–40

Molan P (2005) Mode of action. In: White R, Cooper R, Molan P, eds. *Honey: A modern wound management product*. Wounds UK, Aberdeen

National Institute of Health and Clinical Excellence (2004) *Clinical Guidelines for Type 2 diabetes: prevention and management of foot problems*. NICE, London

Parnham A (2002) Moist wound healing: does the theory apply to chronic wounds? *J Wound Care* **11**(4): 143–6

Schultz GS, Barillo DJ, Moringo DW, Chin GA (2004) Wound bed preparation and a brief history of TIME. *Int Wound J* **1**(1): 19–32

Santos D, Carline T (2000) Examination of the lower limb in high risk patients. *J Tissue Viability* **10**(3): 97–105

Subrahmanyam M (1996) Honey dressing versus boiled potato peel in the treatment of burns: a prospective randomised study. *Burns* **22**(6): 491–3

Vowden K, Vowden P (2004) The role of exudate in the healing process: understanding exudate management. In: White R, ed. *Trends in Wound Care, volume III*. Quay Books, MA Healthcare Ltd, London

Winter GD (1962) Formation of the scab and the rate of epithelialization of superficial wounds in the skin of young domestic pigs. *Nature* **193**: 293–4

Wolf H, Baron R (2003) The theory of pain. In: *Pain at Wound Dressing Changes*. MEP Ltd, London

INDEX

W

X